IMAGES
of America

The Carmelite Sisters for the Aged and Infirm

On the Cover: This photograph taken in 1937 shows the professed sisters, the novices, and the postulants of the Carmelite Sisters for the Aged and Infirm who were serving at St. Patrick's Home in the Bronx, New York. By 1937, the sisters had already opened five different nursing homes—two in Philadelphia and three in New York City. Mother Angeline Teresa McCrory, foundress of the Carmelite Sisters for the Aged and Infirm, is seated in the front row, to the left of the three priests at center. (Courtesy of the Carmelite Sisters for the Aged and Infirm.)

IMAGES
of America

The Carmelite Sisters for the Aged and Infirm

Régine Lambrech and the
Carmelite Sisters for the Aged and Infirm

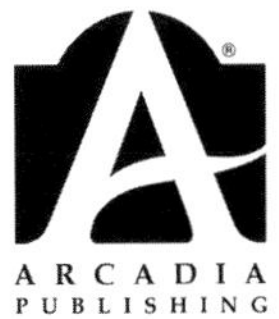
ARCADIA
PUBLISHING

ISBN 978-1-4671-0373-2

Published by Arcadia Publishing
Charleston, South Carolina

Printed in the United States of America

Library of Congress Control Number: 2019934990

For all general information, please contact Arcadia Publishing:
Telephone 843-853-2070
Fax 843-853-0044
E-mail sales@arcadiapublishing.com
For customer service and orders:
Toll-Free 1-888-313-2665

Visit us on the Internet at www.arcadiapublishing.com

This book is dedicated to the legacy of our foundress, Mother M. Angeline Teresa McCrory, and to all the Carmelite Sisters for the Aged and Infirm who have provided, and who continue to provide, loving care to the geriatric patients and residents under their supervision.

Contents

Acknowledgments

The Carmelite Sisters for the Aged and Infirm have been caring for the elderly for over 90 years now. They have been called pioneers in the field of geriatrics, received numerous awards for their work, and introduced person-centered care way before that became the buzzword it is today. Devoted daughters of the church and its teachings, they have continued to be leaders in the care of the elderly since their founding in 1929.

This book would not have come to fruition without the support and encouragement of all the Carmelite Sisters, many of whom shared their stories or their photographs. Their guidance and input have been invaluable to me. I especially wish to thank Mother Mark Louis Anne, who carved time out of her busy schedule to review this manuscript and to help identify some of the sisters in the photographs. Sr. Patricia Queen of Carmel and Sr. Therese Mary also helped to identify some of the older sisters and provided background stories about them. Sr. Christopher Jude patiently printed out many jpgs so we could be sure of the clarity of the images. I would also like to thank Mary Ann Iaccino for her invaluable help in scanning and categorizing the photographs with me as well as for her creative input regarding the layout.

Images for this book, unless otherwise stated, are courtesy of the archives of the Carmelite Sisters for the Aged and Infirm.

—Régine Lambrech
Historian and Archivist
Carmelite Sisters for the Aged and Infirm

Introduction

The Carmelite Sisters for the Aged and Infirm celebrate their 90th year of care for the elderly in 2019. Their story begins with Brigid McCrory, who was born on January 21, 1893, in Mountjoy, Ireland (Northern Ireland since 1921). When she was eight, her family (four children and her parents) moved to Scotland, where her father found work at the Clydesdale Steel Works; a great number of Irish workers were already employed there. The family originally lived in Carfin but moved to Mossend, Bellshill, which was another suburb of Glasgow. Anna, the youngest McCrory child, along with the three other children, had developed measles shortly after the family's arrival in Scotland; Anna did not survive. Brigid and her brother, Owen, and her remaining sister, Liz, attended Holy Family School in Mossend. Brigid left there at the age of 13 to attend the Elmwood Convent School (a high school) in 1906. A year before her graduation, her father was fatally injured in an accident at the Clydesdale Steel Works, where he had been burned by molten steel. Brigid graduated from Elmwood in 1912, having excelled in French, which as we will soon see came in very handy for her.

While Brigid was in school in Scotland, some sisters belonging to the Congregation of the Little Sisters of the Poor came to call regularly on the McCrorys. They were collecting to support a home they ran for the aged poor. At this time, Brigid was discerning a vocation and discussed it with the pastor of her parish, Holy Family Church. The pastor, Father Cronin, encouraged her and supported her decision to enter the Little Sisters of the Poor in Glasgow. She left home on February 2, 1912, to enter the sisters' home there. Six months later, on August 11, 1912, she was sent to the home of the Little Sisters in Paris. Here, Brigid and the other women who entered at the same time were expected to perfect their knowledge of the French language. Clearly, Brigid had a head start and was happy to help the other women feel more confident in the language. The group remained in Paris until February 14, 1913, when the women traveled to the motherhouse of the Little Sisters of the Poor in La Tour St. Joseph. She received her habit and her religious name of Sr. Marie Angeline de Ste Agathe on September 8, 1913.

During her novitiate at La Tour St. Joseph, she participated in the care of the aged, since the older sisters were assigned to the hospital care of the French soldiers returning from the nearby battlefields of World War I. This time spent as a novice allowed Sr. Marie Angeline's spirituality to develop, and she loved the ceremonies organized for the various church feasts. She read French spiritual writers and years later quoted many of them in the circular letters she sent to the Carmelite Sisters. On March 19, 1915, she pronounced her first vows as a Little Sister of the Poor but could not go to her first assignment at St. Augustine's Home in Brooklyn, New York, due to the war and the dangers of traveling by ship. Finally, she and several other Little Sisters of the Poor left the motherhouse on October 15, 1915, and arrived in New York on October 31.

It was in New York that Sr. Marie Angeline developed her lifelong love of America and the American people. Many of the residents of St. Augustine's Home were immigrants themselves but had adapted to the American way of life. They contributed to the functioning of the home by using their talents since they were alone and poor, but not as acutely ill as many of the residents in nursing homes today.

In addition to caring for the elderly residents, Sr. Marie Angeline was sent out to beg for alms from the general public. In September 1919, at the age of 26, she was appointed by the motherhouse of the Little Sisters in France to be a councillor and to assist the local mother superior in the running of the St. Augustine Home. She was also given responsibility for some of the internal affairs of the Little Sisters operating the Brooklyn home. It had to have been highly unusual for the French order to confide such responsibilities to a young Irish sister.

After nine years in New York, she was recalled to the motherhouse in France to prepare for her perpetual vows, which she pronounced on April 21, 1925. While most congregations pronounce the three vows of poverty, chastity, and obedience, the Little Sisters of the Poor add a fourth vow of hospitality. She was then missioned to Pittsburgh in May 1925. Less than three months later, in August 1925, she was named assistant superior of the home there. Only a little more than a year later, in August 1926, Sr. Marie Angeline was named mother superior of Our Lady's Home in the Bronx and assumed this new role on October 7, 1926. She was only 33 years of age at the time and took on the responsibility for 18 sisters and 230 elderly residents.

Stepping into her new role, she began to look for ways to serve the needs of her "old people." She saw an unmet need in America—care for the elderly who had a bit of money but no one to look after them in their old age. She also wished to make the accommodations of the residents more homelike, allow married couples to share a room, if able, and celebrate American holidays such as Thanksgiving. As an attempt to restore order after the chaos of World War I, the superior general of the Little Sisters at the time endeavored to keep all Little Sisters' homes in full conformity to the standard of living and care of the elderly in France. This mandate immediately presented a conundrum for the sisters at Our Lady's Home because it placed them at odds with two of their vows. If they followed the dictates of the superior general they would disobey their vow of hospitality, and if they continued with their desire to serve the elderly of all incomes according to the standards of America, they were not respecting their vow of obedience. Mother Angeline turned to her confessor, Fr. Edwin Sinnott, who advised her to go see Cardinal Hayes, head of the Archdiocese of New York. Since she was a bit shy about approaching the cardinal, Father Sinnott prepared the way for her. When she met with the cardinal and explained the situation to him, he assured her that he would do everything he could to assist her and that she had made the right decision to come forward to present the conditions to him. As a result, the cardinal sent Bishop John Dunn to make a canonical visit to Our Lady's Home on January 15, 1929. He also visited the other two homes in New York sponsored by the Little Sisters and noted similar circumstances.

On June 19, 1929, Bishop Dunn visited Our Lady's Home for a second time, during the visit of Mother Gertrude, assistant to the mother general. Mother Angeline and six other sisters spoke to the bishop in the presence of Mother Gertrude. The seven sisters informed Bishop Dunn of their desire to be dispensed of their vows as Little Sisters but not to leave the religious life. They sent their written request for dispensation to Rome on June 21, the requests arrived on August 5, and they were signed in Rome on August 9, 1929. Mother Angeline and her six companions left the Little Sisters on August 11, 1929, and were welcomed by the Sparkill Dominicans at their convent of St. Martin of Tours Parish in the Bronx. Leaving with her were Sisters Louise, of Belgium; Leonie, of Boston; Colette, of Ireland; Mary Teresa, of Richmond, Virginia; and Alodie and Alexis, of Canada.

Less than a month later, on September 3, 1929, the seven sisters, through the efforts of Cardinal Hayes, moved into the old rectory of St. Elizabeth's Parish in New York City. To this day, the Carmelite Sisters for the Aged and Infirm celebrate September 3 as Foundation Day. At St. Elizabeth's on October 29, 1929, four days after the American stock market crashed, Mother Angeline and her six companion sisters took in their first four elderly residents. Support came from Catholic Charities and donations of vestments, a chalice, and a ciborium. Crucifixes for each of the sisters' rooms came from various priest friends. It was a tremendous leap of faith to set out to serve the elderly right at the start of the Great Depression when money was so very tight.

Mother Angeline felt the desire for herself and her six other sisters to be affiliated with one of the great orders of the church. She enlisted the help of the Very Reverend Lawrence Flanagan, O. Carm., the provincial of the New York Province of the Carmelites, who had been an early supporter of Mother Angeline. In fact, while she was still at Our Lady's Home, it was Father Flanagan who brought Mother Angeline a bouquet of roses on the feast of St. Thérèse of the Child Jesus on October 3, 1928. To this day, the Carmelite Sisters for the Aged and Infirm keep up this Carmelite tradition and distribute roses on St. Thérèse's feast day.

Father Flanagan was instrumental in advising Mother Angeline to see Cardinal Hayes to make her request for his permission to be affiliated with the Ancient Order of Carmel. In early April 1931, Mother Angeline met with Cardinal Hayes and followed that visit with a letter dated April 15, 1931, thanking the cardinal for his many kindnesses and telling him that each of the seven sisters was more than satisfied with the name "Carmelite Sisters for the Aged and Infirm" and that they were anxious to be affiliated with the Carmelite order. Approval from the cardinal arrived on June 22, 1931, and the personal involvement of the Most Reverend Elias Magennis, O. Carm., prior general of the Carmelite order, allowed the sisters to obtain rapid approval from Rome. The actual date of the reception of the Carmelite affiliation was July 16, 1931, the feast of Our Lady of Mount Carmel, and thus the sisters became the first congregation in America to be dedicated solely to the care of the aging.

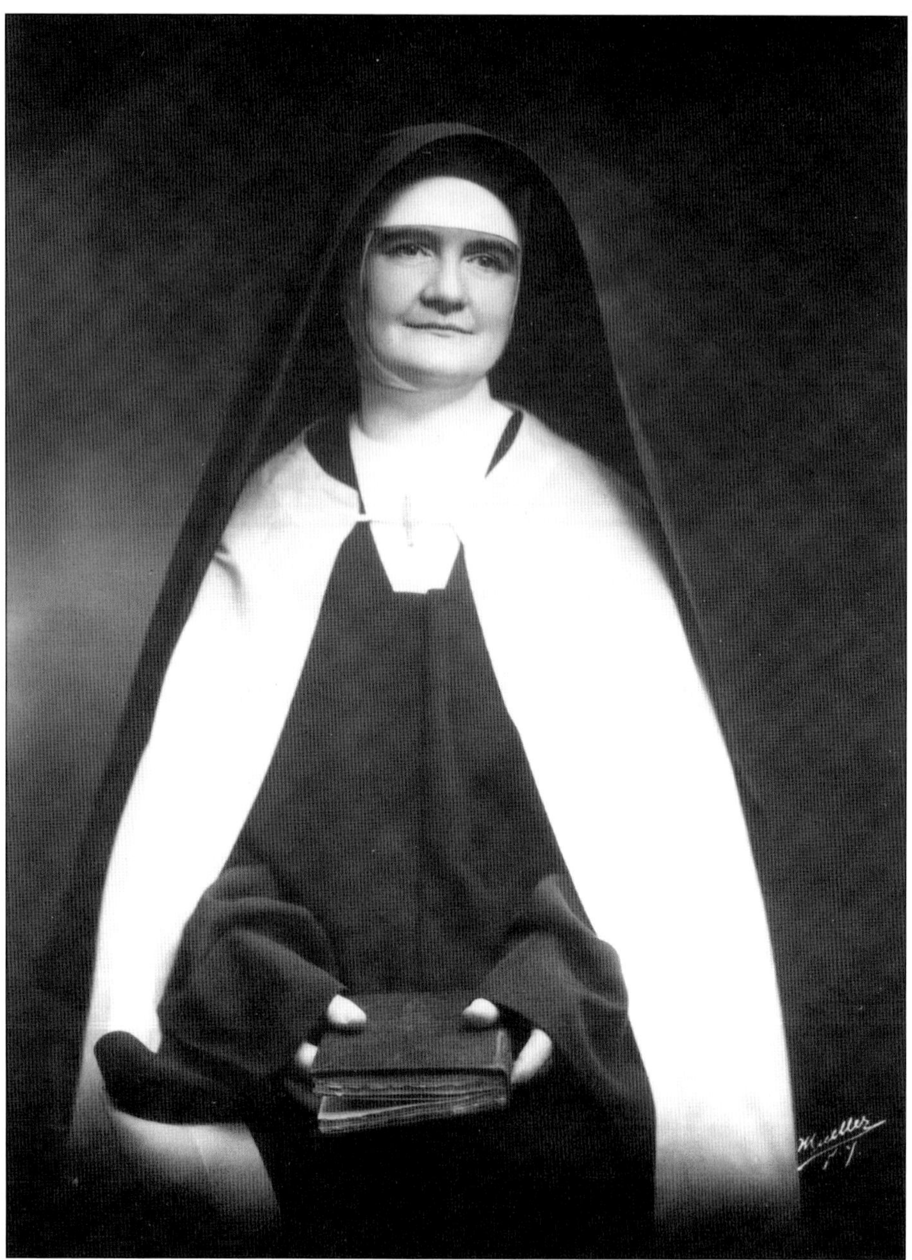

Born on January 21, 1893, in Mountjoy, Ireland, Brigid Teresa McCrory entered the Little Sisters of the Poor in Glasgow in 1912. Her family had moved to Scotland where her father had found work in the Clydesdale Steel factory. Upon her profession of first vows at the Little Sisters' motherhouse in France, she was sent to the United States to work in nursing homes. In September 1929, she founded a new congregation in New York, the Carmelite Sisters for the Aged and Infirm, dedicated to serving elderly middle-class Americans who had no one to care for them. She took the name of Sr. M. Angeline Teresa, O.Carm. At the age of 36, she was named the first superior general and was continually reelected as superior general until she stepped down in 1978. Mother Angeline was declared venerable by Pope Benedict XVI in July 2012. This portrait of her was taken by Mueller Photography in 1936 in New York.

One

Founding of the Community and Early Days, 1929–1947

The Little Sisters of the Poor took in only the destitute in the early years of the 20th century. At that time in the city of New York, there were many middle-class Americans who had no one to take care of them in their old age. Sr. Angeline de Ste Agathe, as administrator of the home of the Little Sisters of the Poor, Our Lady's Home in the Bronx, felt awful that so many needy elderly persons were being turned away because they had "too much" money.

In August 1929, Sr. Angeline Teresa and six other Little Sisters of the Poor left their order under the protection of Cardinal Hayes of New York. For a short time, they lived with the Dominican Sisters from Sparkill, New York, who had a convent at St. Martin of Tours in New York City. The cardinal then gave the sisters an unused rectory from St. Elizabeth's Parish and they took in their first seven residents.

On July 12, 1931, they received permission from Rome to call themselves the Carmelite Sisters for the Aged and Infirm; Cardinal Hayes named Mother Angeline superior general of the new order. On August 15, 1931, Cardinal Hayes bought them a building in the Bronx, which they named St. Patrick's Home. One month later, the sisters and their residents moved into the new home, which also served as a convent, novitiate, and nursing home.

Four years later, they added three more floors to the facility to welcome more elderly persons, and the numbers of sisters and residents steadily grew. By the time that the community outgrew the convent and novitiate at St. Patrick's, and Mother Angeline purchased property in Germantown, New York, in December 1946 to move the motherhouse there, she had opened 12 nursing homes and had sisters serving in seven seminaries.

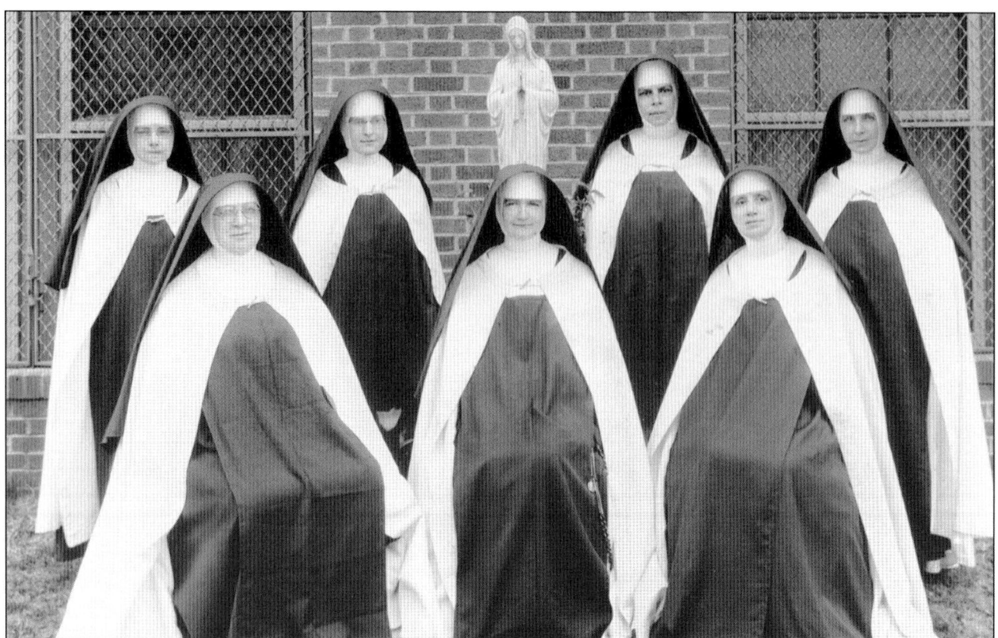

This is an extremely rare photograph of all seven original Carmelite sisters together (all former Little Sisters of the Poor). From left to right are (first row) Mother Louise, Mother Angeline Teresa, and Mother Leonie; (second row) Mother Alodie, Mother Alexis, Mother Teresa, and Mother Colette. They welcomed their first elderly residents to the former St. Elizabeth's Rectory in the Bronx in 1929.

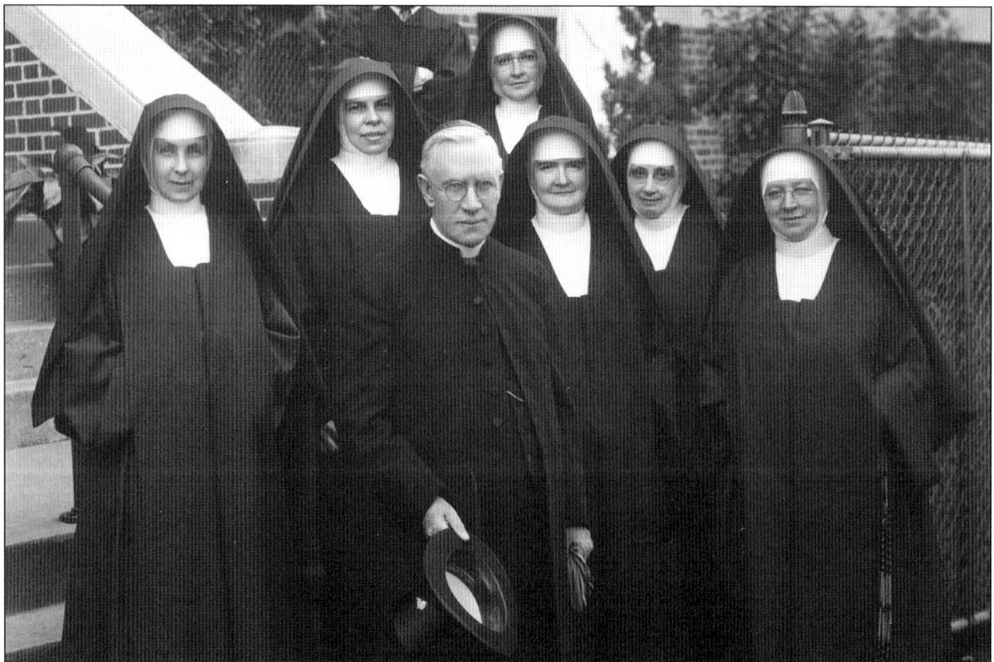

Patrick Cardinal Hayes is seen here in front of St. Patrick's Home with Mother Angeline and four of the original six sisters who left the Little Sisters of the Poor with her. This photograph was taken by Mueller Photography in 1931.

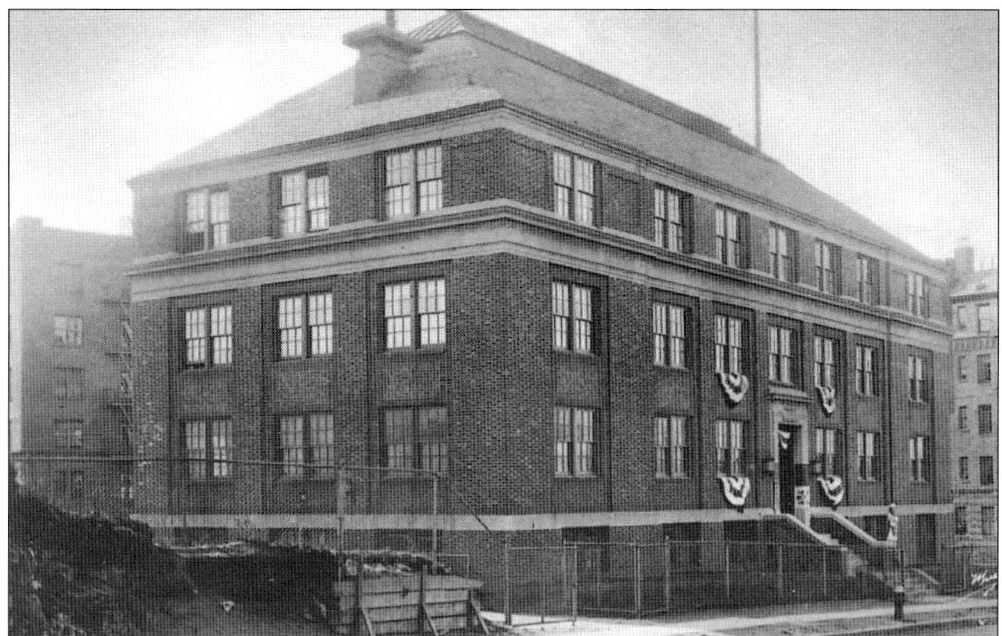

This is the original St. Patrick's Home as it appeared in 1931, when the building was acquired from RCA. Partly visible on the roof are the radio antennae that received the first transatlantic radio broadcast from London to New York City in 1924. Work was immediately undertaken to convert it into a nursing home with individual rooms for residents, rooms for the sisters, dining rooms, and a chapel. Permission to print this photograph from *A Call to Care* © 1996 was granted by the Catholic Health Association of the United States.

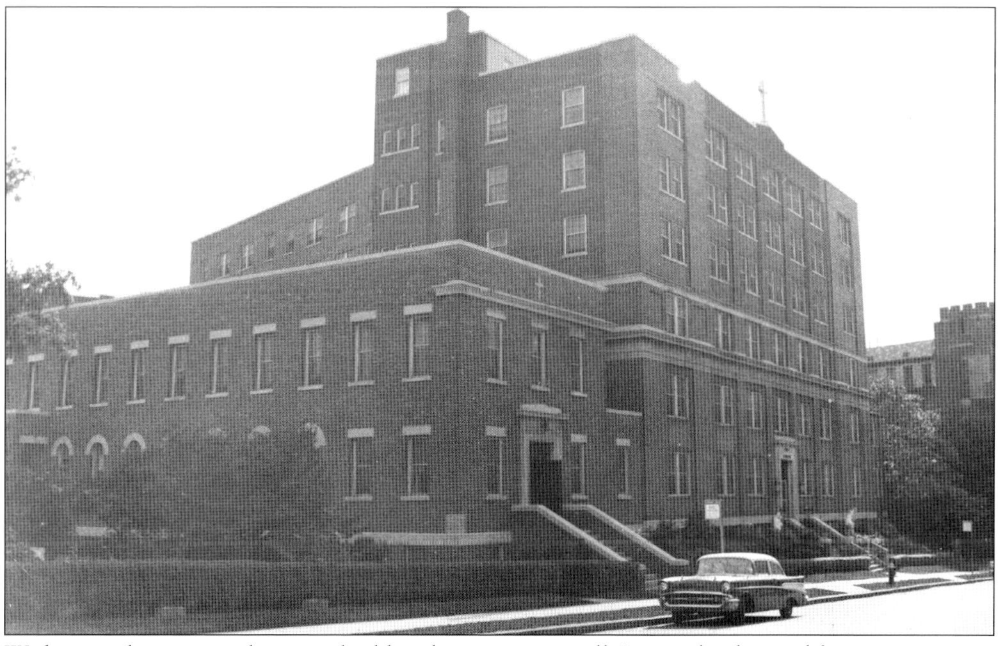

Within six short years, this same building became too small. Just as the demand for rooms grew, so did the number of vocations. The building underwent the construction of a three-story addition in 1936 and a separate novitiate for postulants and novices.

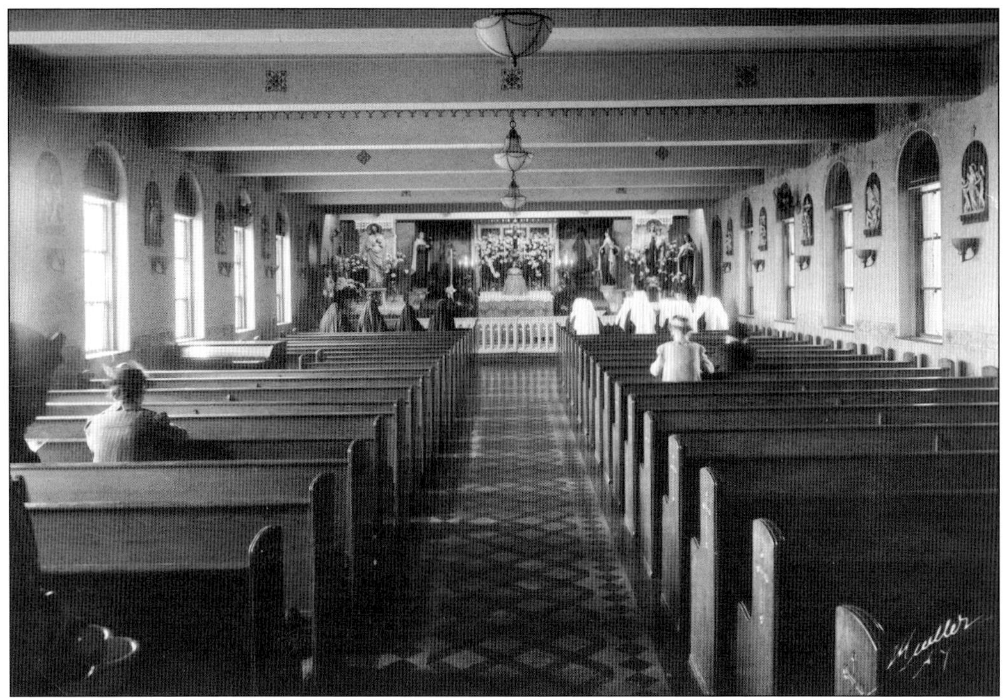

The original chapel in St. Patrick's Home had room for 125 residents and sisters. To the left of the altar is the painting of St. Patrick and to the right is that of Ste Thérèse, the Little Flower. This undated photograph was taken by Mueller Photography.

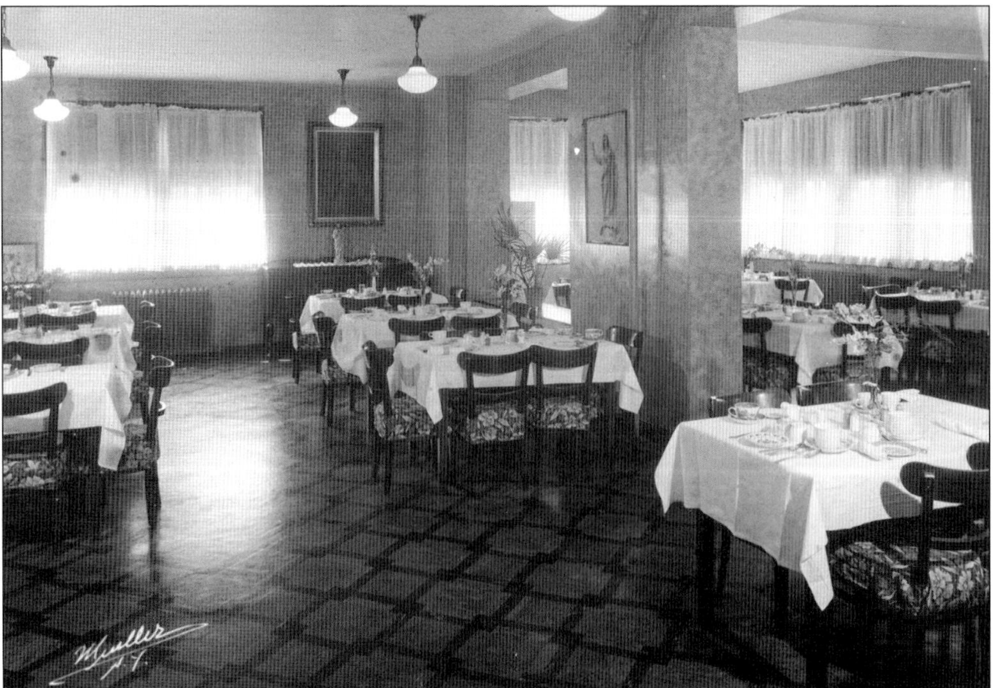

This is one of the early dining rooms for residents. The tables were always set with tablecloths, china, glassware, and cutlery—nothing but the best for the residents.

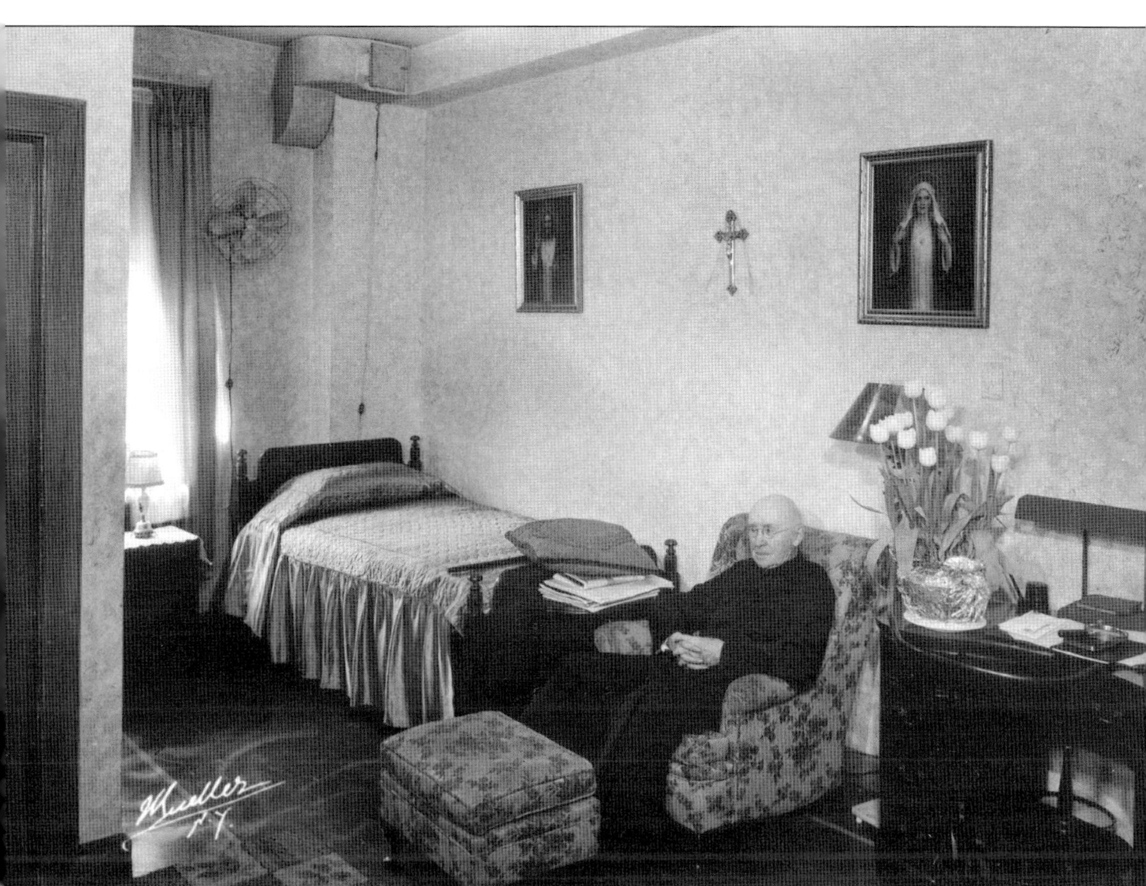

Father Cunion, a retired priest, can be seen in his room at St. Patrick's Home in this photograph taken in 1940. He had served at St. Rita of Cascia Parish in the Bronx before taking up residency at St. Patrick's Home. This undated photograph was taken by Mueller Photography.

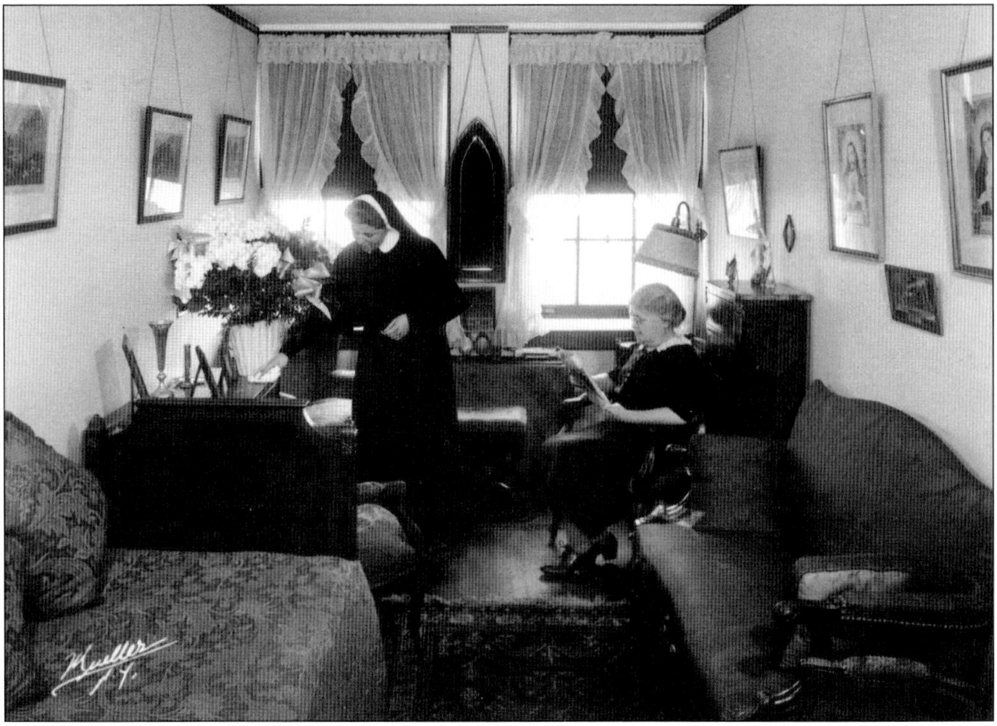

A postulant dusts the room of a resident who is surrounded by furniture that the sisters encouraged her to bring from home so that her room would truly reflect her own belongings and personality.

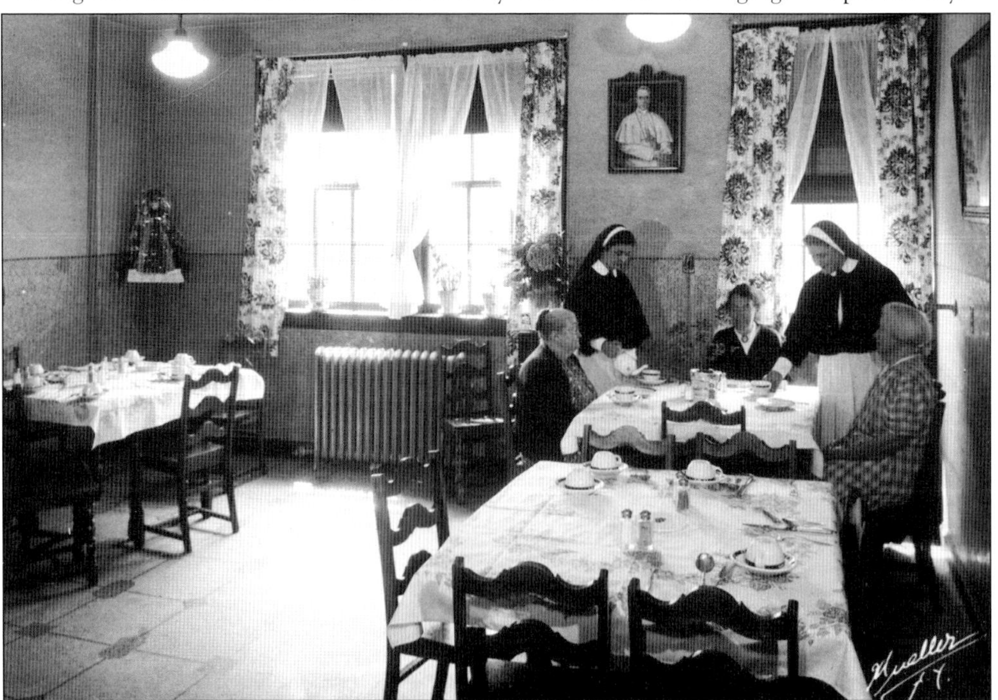

Two postulants are serving a meal to residents in another of the early dining rooms at St. Patrick's Home. This undated photograph was taken by Mueller Photography.

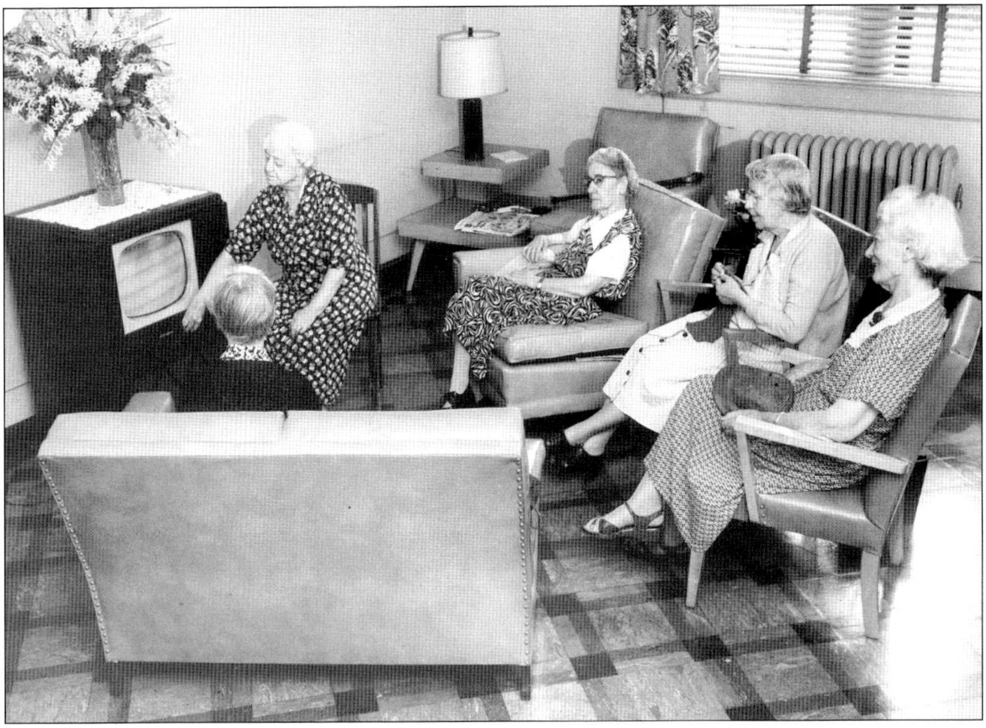

In one of the common rooms, female residents gather around an early television set as it warms up.

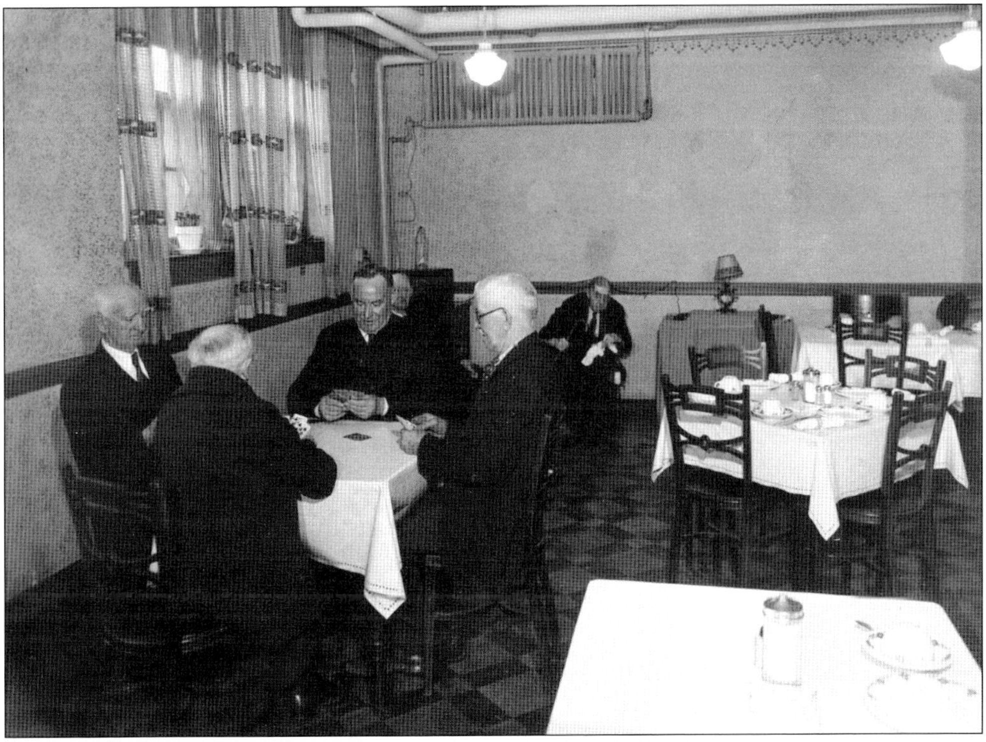

Some of the male residents stay behind to play cards after the lunch meal.

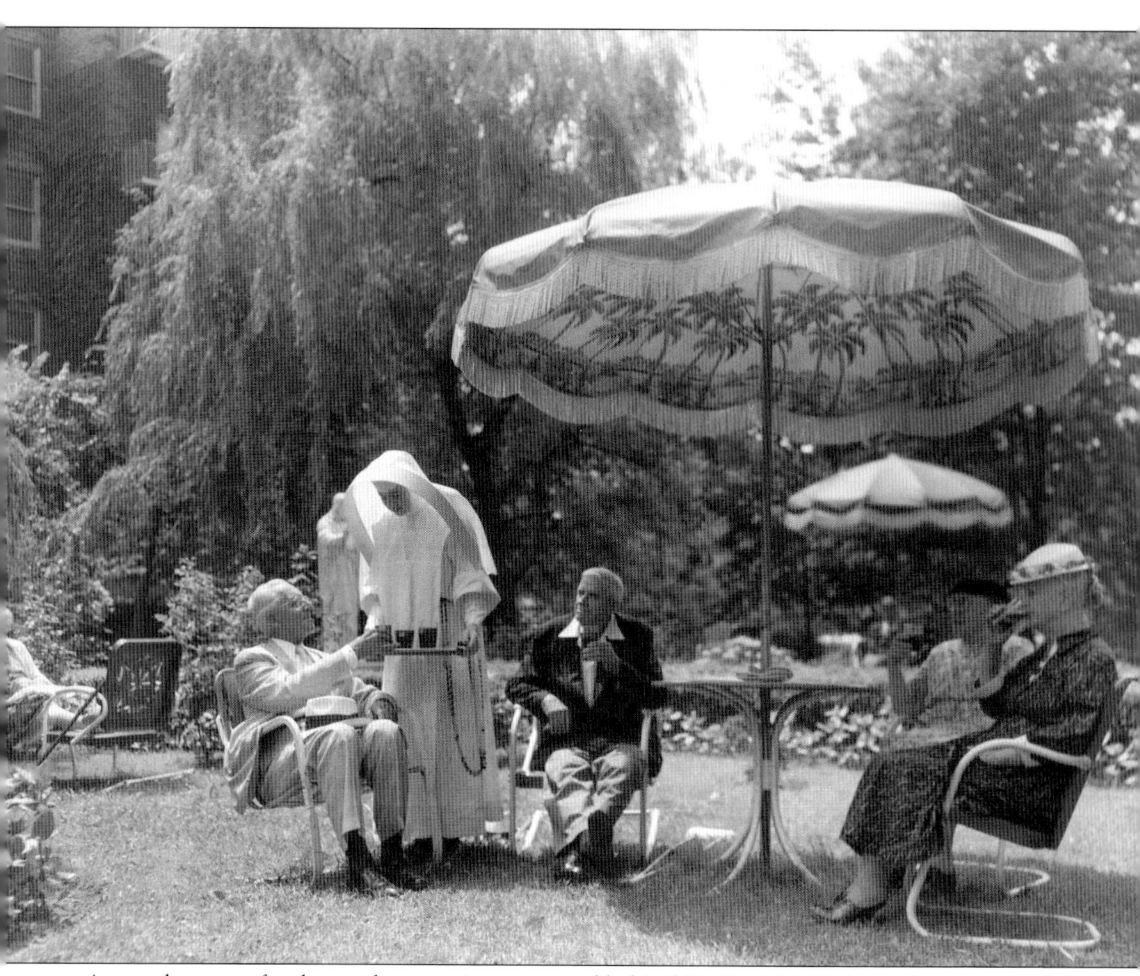

An outdoor area for the residents to sit was created behind St. Patrick's Home and was especially appreciated by those who were unable to cross the street to use Van Cortlandt Park. A sister can be seen serving residents a beverage.

This is the first novitiate building at St. Patrick's Home. It was a converted garage enlarged to accommodate two floors of dormitory-like rooms for the postulants and novices.

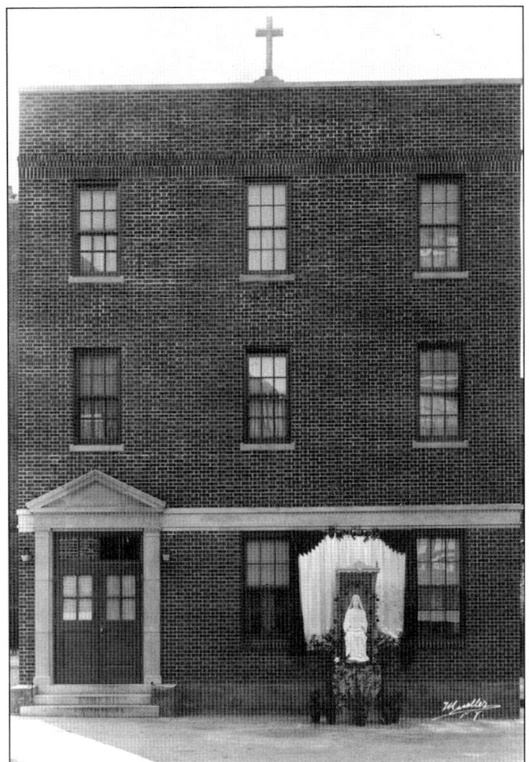

This is one of the dormitories. Each sister had a bed and a locker separated from the next by a curtain. This undated photograph was taken by Mueller Photography.

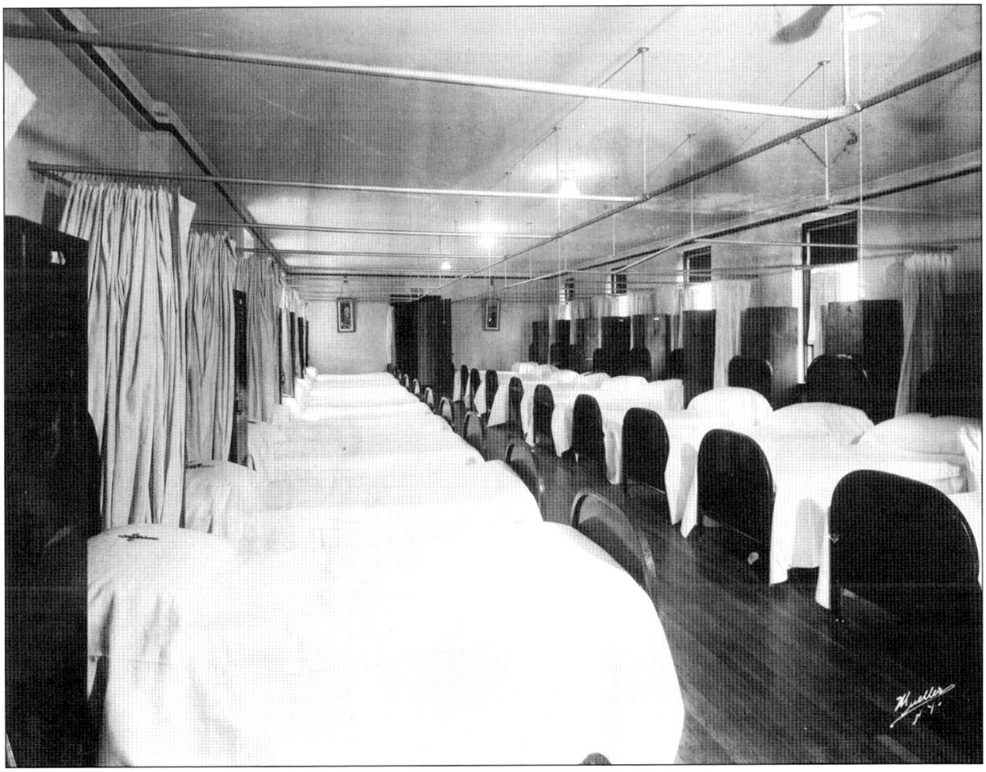

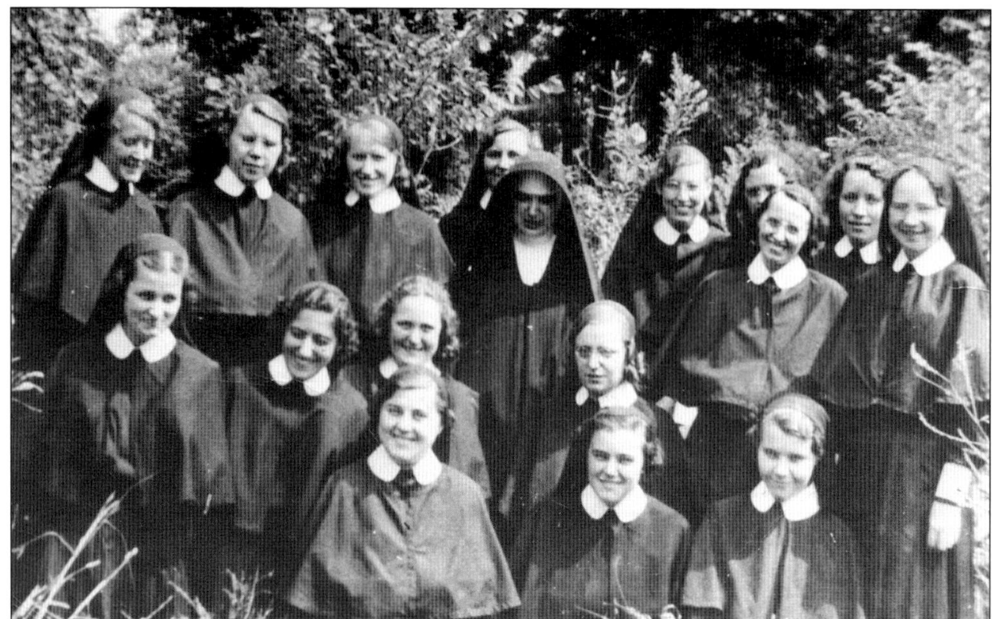

In this undated photograph, Sr. Bernadette de Lourdes can be seen with a group of postulants wearing the earliest postulant dress.

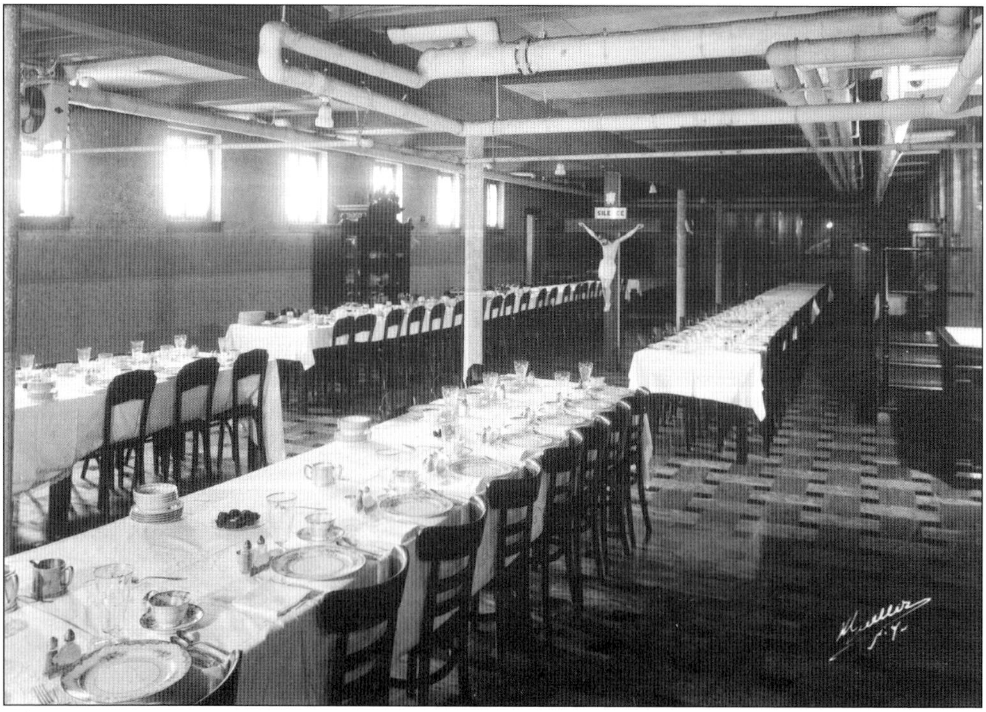

This is the refectory (dining room) for the professed sisters and the novices and postulants in the basement of St. Patrick's Home.

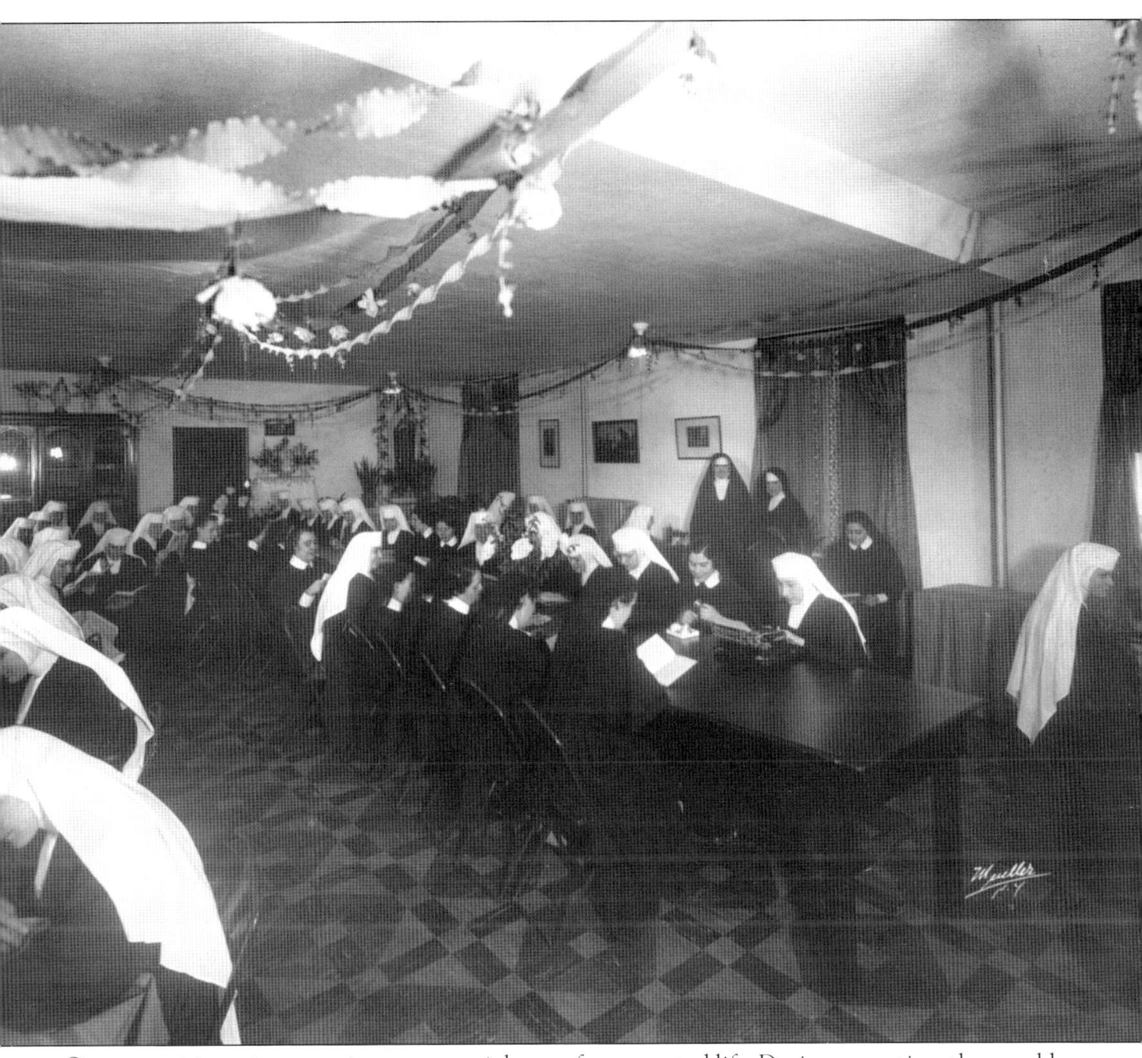

Sisters participate in recreation, an essential part of consecrated life. During recreation, they could sew, knit, sing, get to know each other, and enjoy the beauty of community life. This photograph was taken by Mueller Photography.

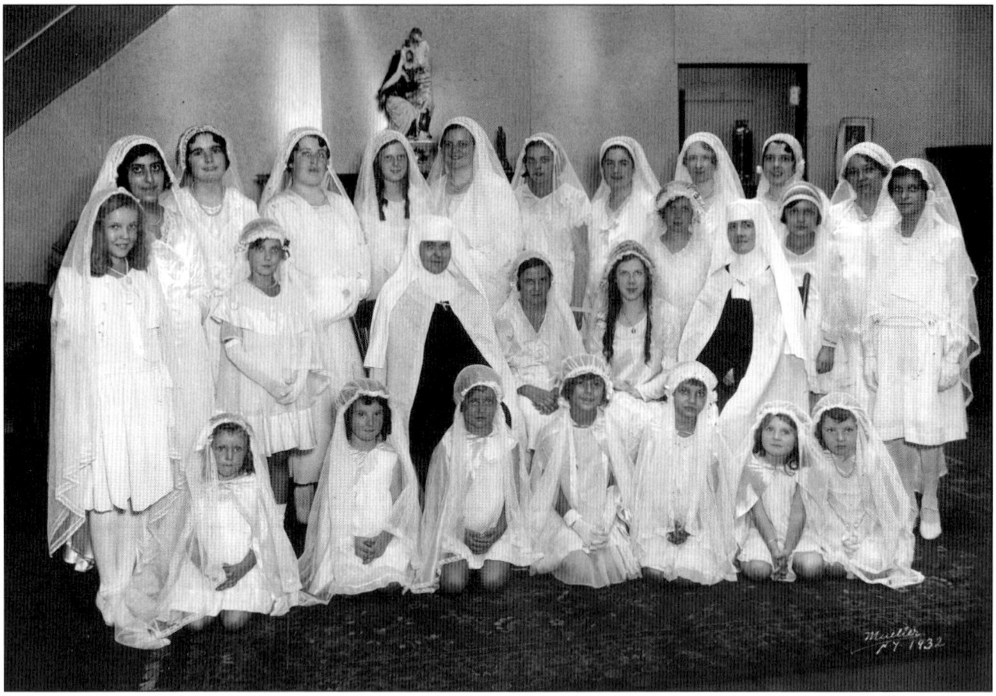

This is a Mueller Photography picture dated September 12, 1932, of the reception of the third group of postulants entering the novitiate. In the early days, bridal gowns were worn by the women. Little girls who had made their communion recently were part of the ceremony and served as flower girls.

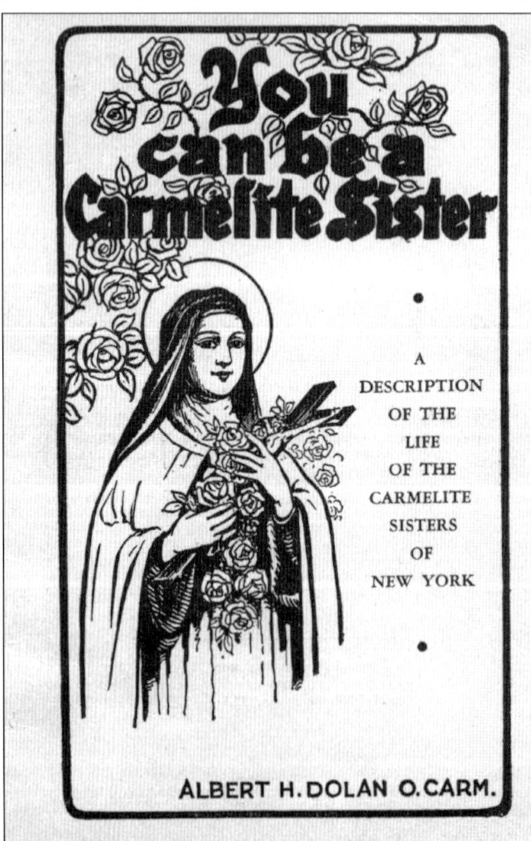

You can be a Carmelite Sister

A DESCRIPTION OF THE LIFE OF THE CARMELITE SISTERS OF NEW YORK

ALBERT H. DOLAN O.CARM.

The sisters had vocational booklets printed, and distributed them to young women they thought might be interested in becoming sisters and serving the elderly. Fr. Albert Dolan, O.Carm., wrote this booklet for the Carmelite Sisters in 1938.

Two

Expansion of the Community and Its Facilities

Vocations increased as many young high school girls came in contact with the sisters serving in various facilities across the country. These young girls volunteered at the nursing homes as Carmelettes, and many later entered the community. Mother Angeline wanted a proper chapel, and in 1952, five years after moving the motherhouse to Germantown, a new chapel was built and blessed.

The novitiate then grew too small, and two years after the construction of the chapel, a new novitiate building was built with room for 75 novices; it also included classrooms and reception rooms. Since the sisters all make an annual retreat at the motherhouse, a five-story retreat house with 60 individual rooms was built and blessed in 1961. In 1967, a private wing was constructed for visiting priests, along with Carmel Hall, a multipurpose assembly hall and gymnasium with a stage and large kitchen. In 1980, the Teresian Library was dedicated; it holds reference and technical books along with periodicals on theology, spirituality, gerontology, and geriatrics.

At the same time, bishops from around the country reached out to Mother Angeline to ask her to either build a facility in their dioceses or to take over a building and convert it into a nursing home. By the time she died in 1984, sisters were serving or had served in 59 different facilities or seminaries. Only a few of those facilities are pictured in the following pages. In several cases, the original facility is pictured and beneath that is a photograph of the facility as it was modernized or enlarged.

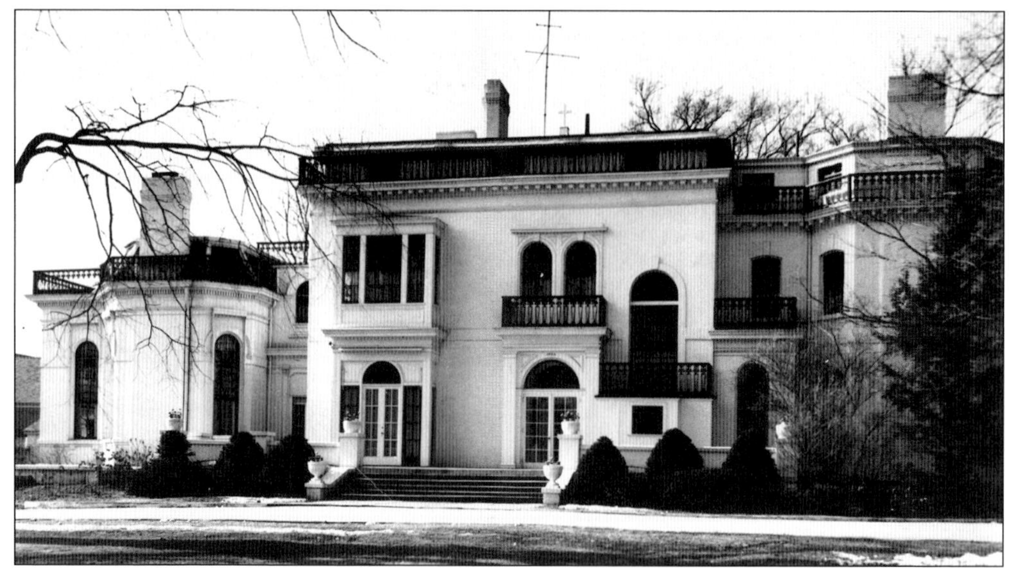

When the congregation outgrew the novitiate at Saint Patrick's Home, Mother Angeline set out to find a suitable location to allow for the expansion of the numbers of young women entering the community. An 86-acre estate on the Hudson River was for sale, and she acquired it in December 1946. This is the front of the home on the property as it looked when it was acquired. On the left is a room that was a library; it was promptly turned into a chapel.

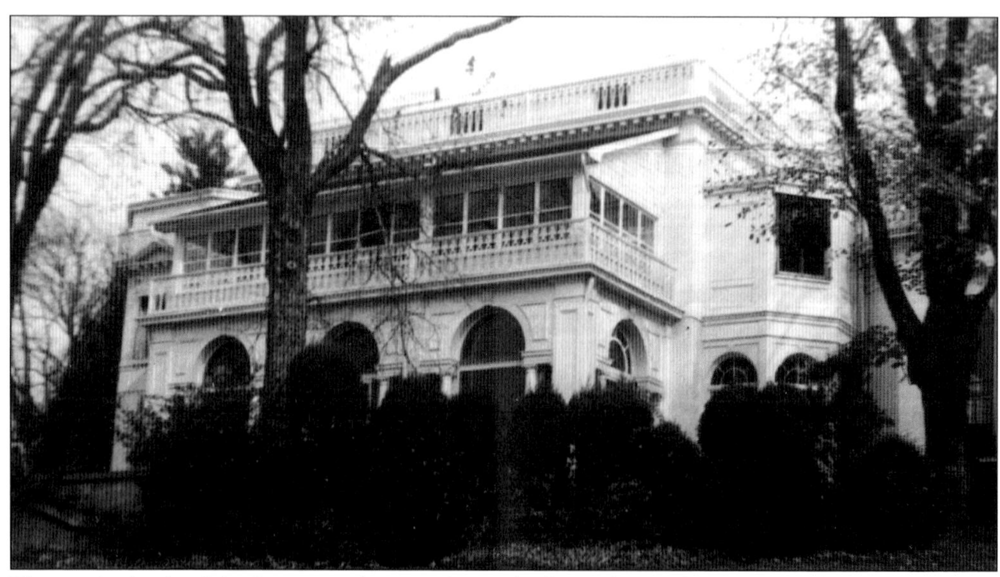

This is the back of the house, with a porch overlooking the Hudson River. The sisters refer to this house as the "White House," and it is the motherhouse of the Carmelite Sisters for the Aged and Infirm.

DEUS CHARITAS EST
Je reviendrai
sur la terre
pour faire aimer
L'AMOUR

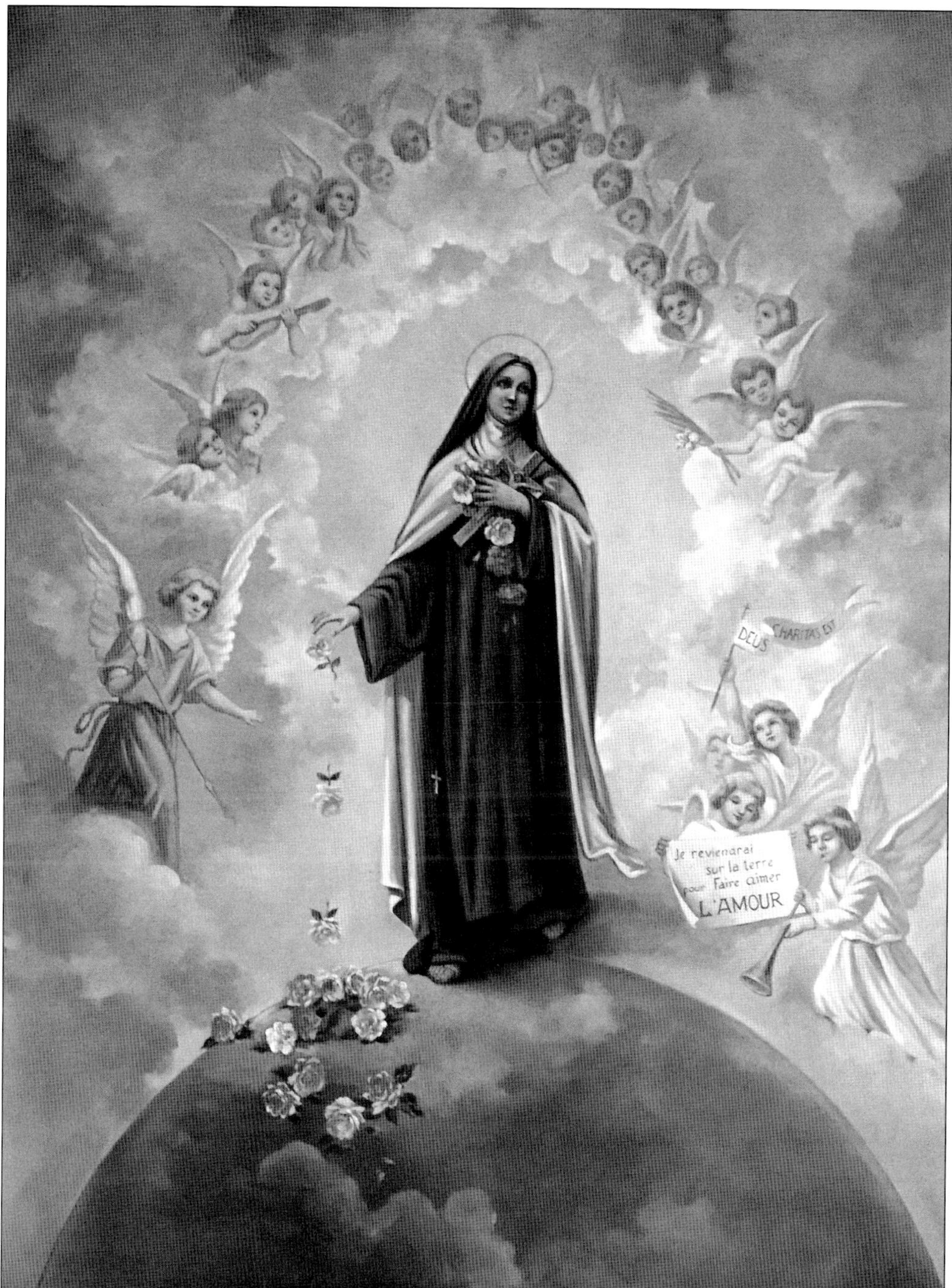

This is the original painting of Ste Thérèse of the Child Jesus that was executed by her sister, Céline, also a Carmelite. Hanging in the entrance hall to the White House, it is eight feet wide by ten feet high. Rev. Albert Dolan, O.Carm., had asked Céline to do the painting when he was promoting the cause of Ste Thérèse in the United States. He gave the painting to Mother Angeline in 1945; she had it mounted on the wall for the dedication of the motherhouse on February 11, 1947.

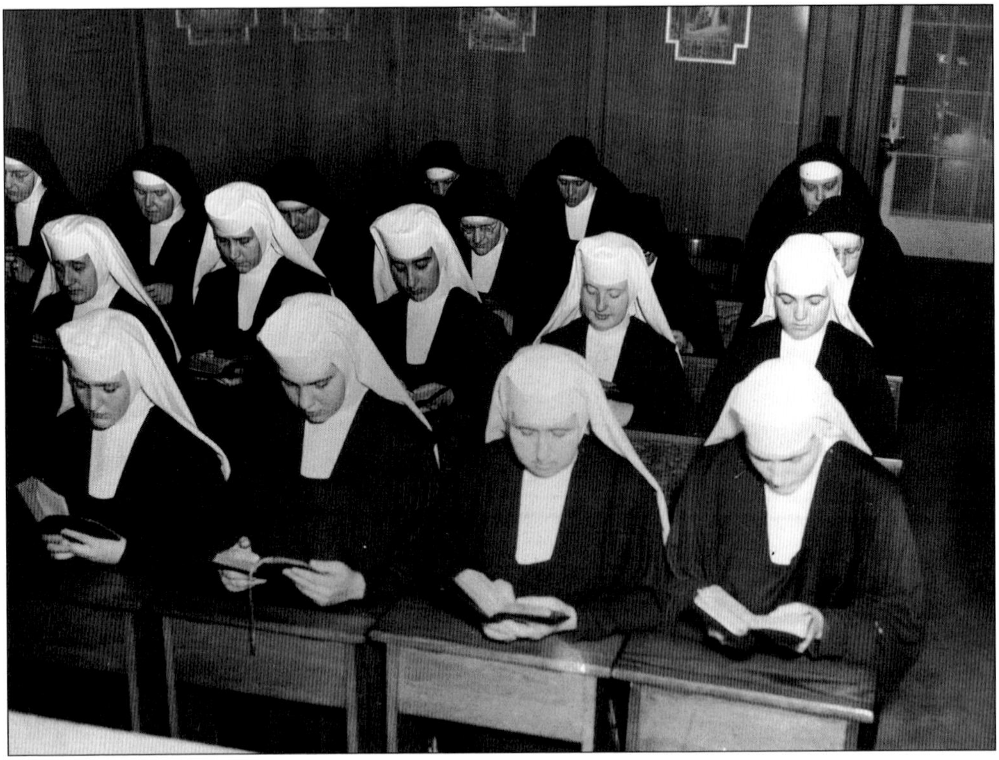

Professed sisters and novices are praying in the first chapel of the motherhouse, which had been converted from the library of the newly acquired home.

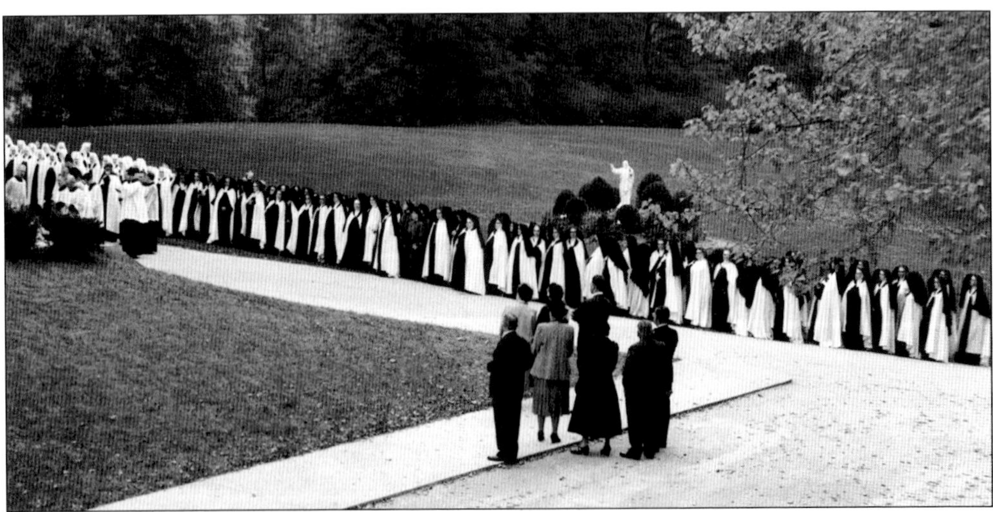

As the congregation grew, the processions increased in size. Here, the professed sisters are forming a welcoming committee as the novices about to make their First Profession process into the chapel for the ceremony. Some family members can be seen in the foreground.

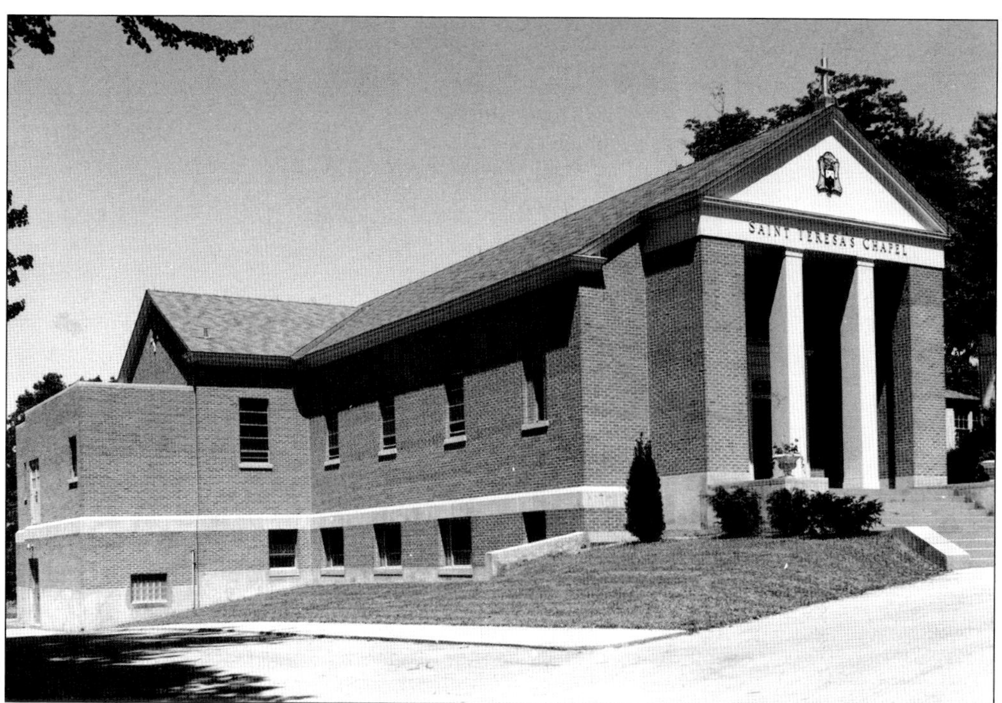

On October 15, 1952, the new chapel pictured here was dedicated to Saint Teresa of Avila. Mother Angeline's cherished dream had come true and another milestone in the community's growth was marked.

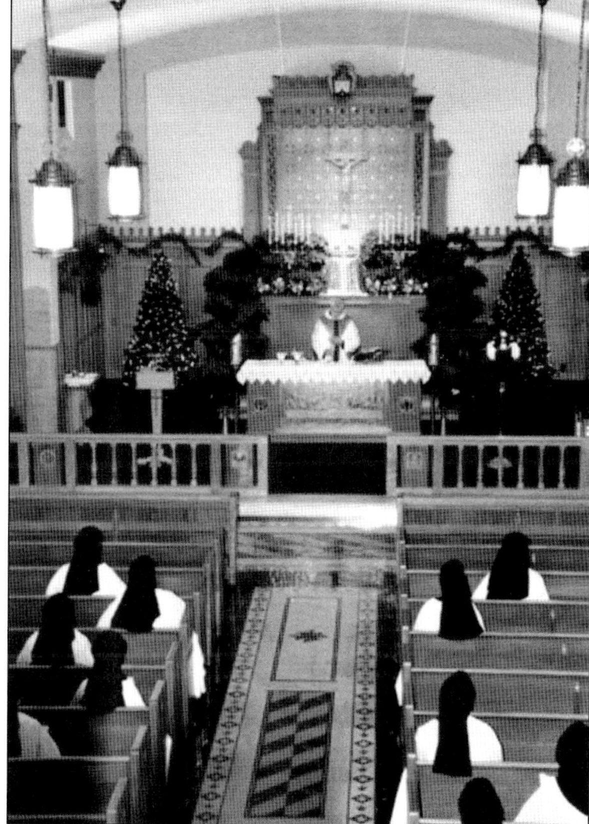

This is the inside of the chapel, which seats 198. The altar front is a beautiful scene of the Last Supper that was hand-carved in Oberammergau, Germany.

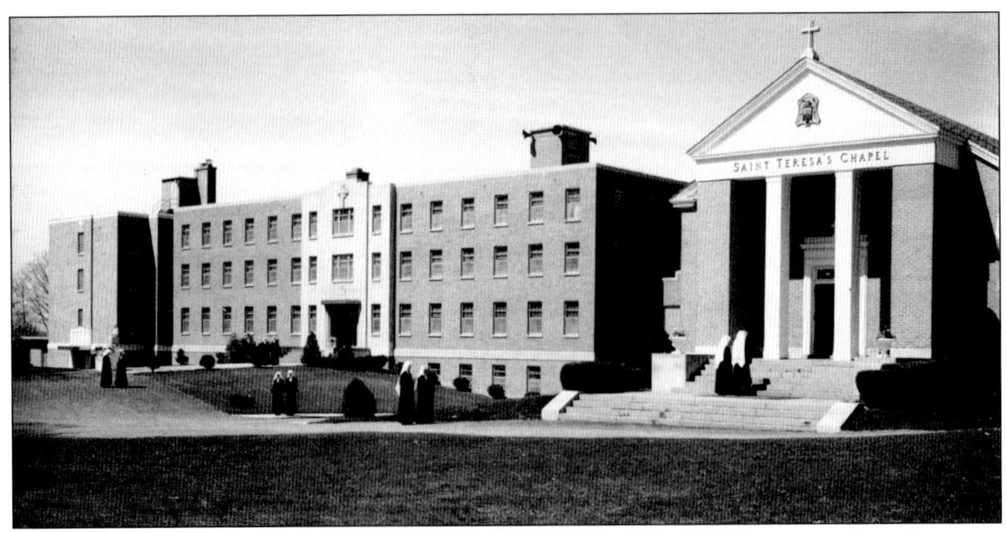

The next endeavor was to build a novitiate to accommodate the increasing number of novices. On November 1, 1954, a brick building was constructed next to the chapel; it featured 75 private rooms, reception rooms, classrooms, and parlors. It was dedicated to Ste Thérèse, the Little Flower.

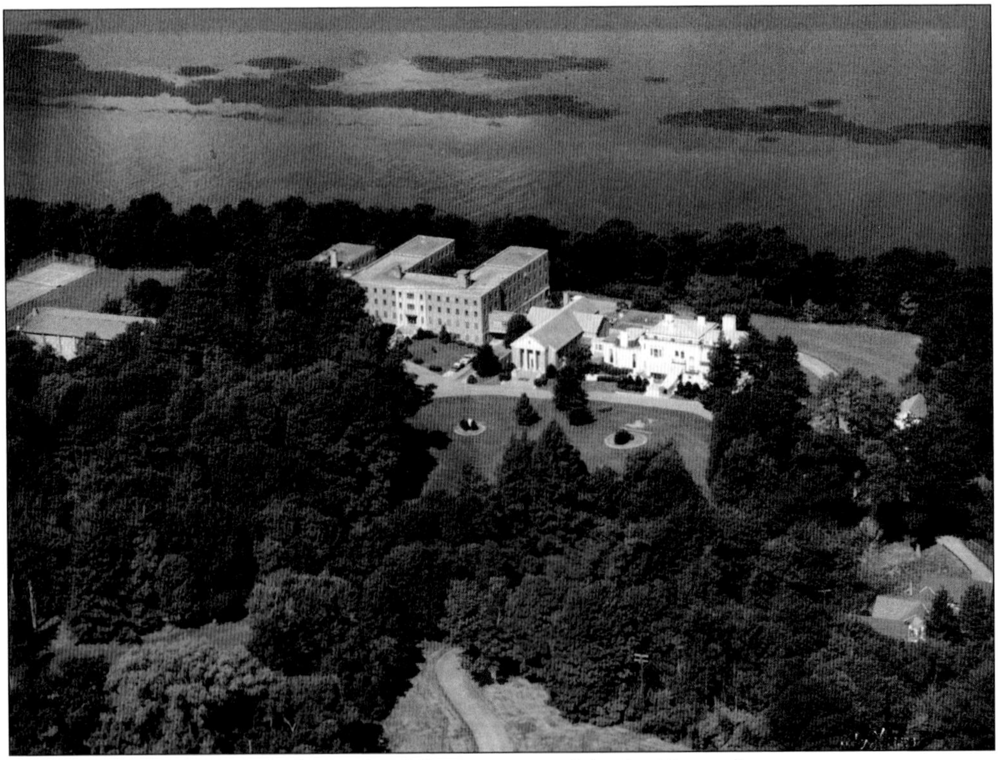

This overhead photograph shows the full expansion of the buildings that span across a quarter mile of frontage on the Hudson River.

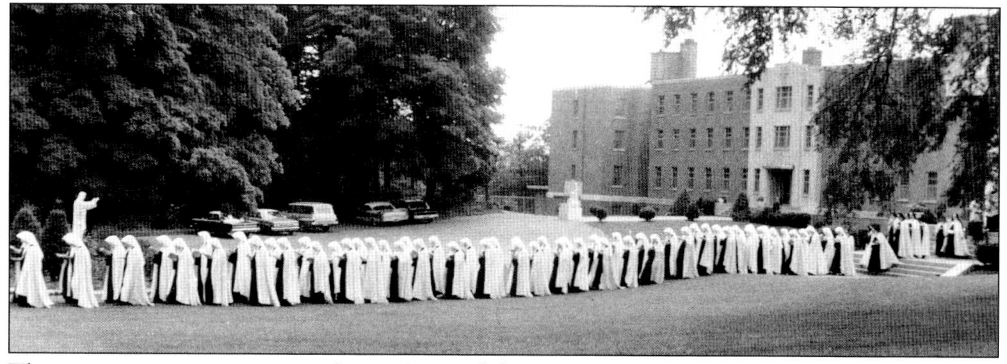

The growing congregation made good use of the new novitiate. Here, a procession of novices leaves the chapel for the feast of Corpus Christi. They processed to three altars set up on the lawn in front of the motherhouse.

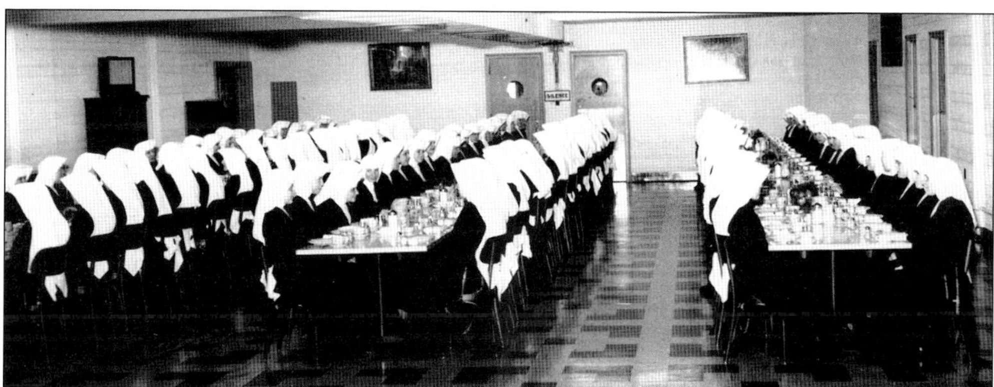

This photograph of the refectory at Avila shows the long tables at which the novices ate. The professed sisters sat at the head of the room at a large U-shaped table. Most meals were taken in silence, with a sister positioned at a lectern to read spiritual writings to the assembly.

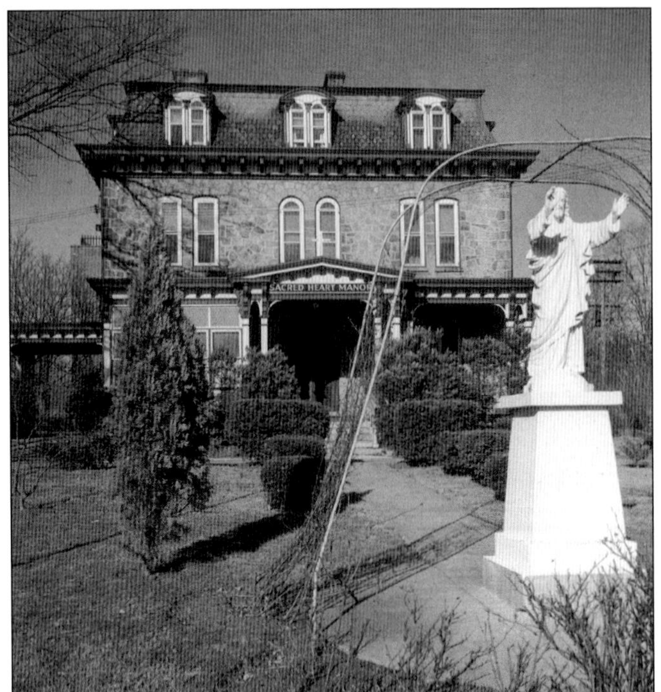

Sacred Heart Manor in Germantown, Pennsylvania, was acquired by the sisters in September 1937; it took one month to get the buildings and surroundings in shape for the dedication ceremony, which took place in October 1937. The first administrator was Mother Alodie, one of the seven sisters who left the Little Sisters of the Poor with Mother Angeline to form the new congregation.

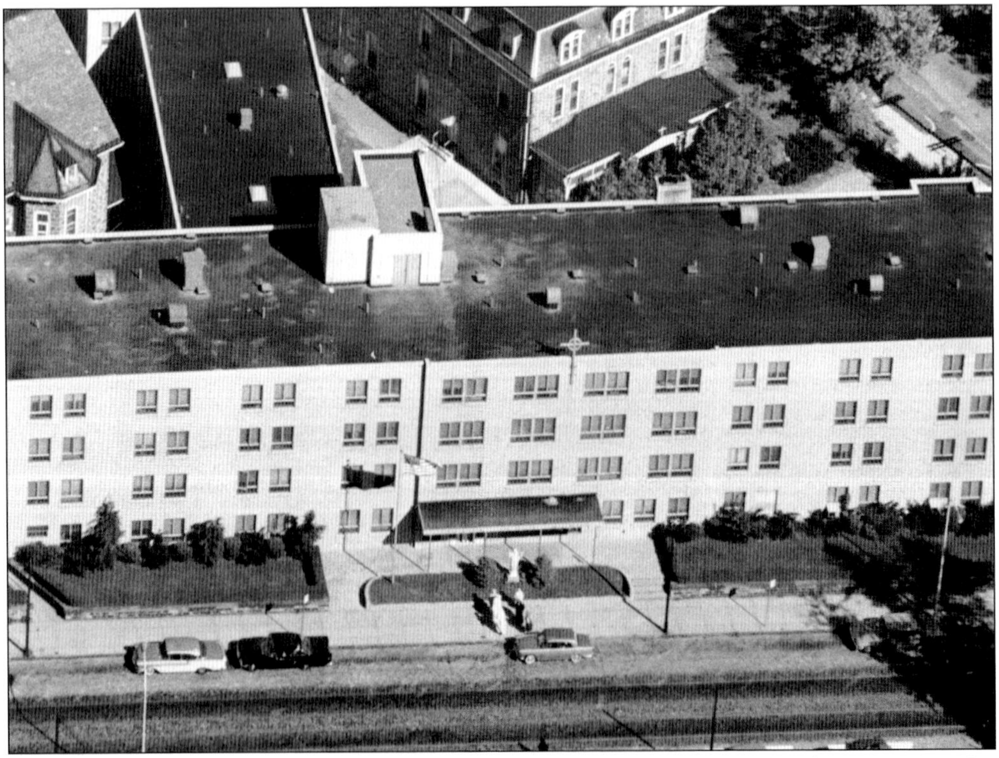

By 1955, a larger home was needed due to the large number of applicants for admission. On May 4, 1957, a new four-story building was blessed by John Cardinal O'Hara, and 140 residents made their home there. The original home can be seen behind the new addition.

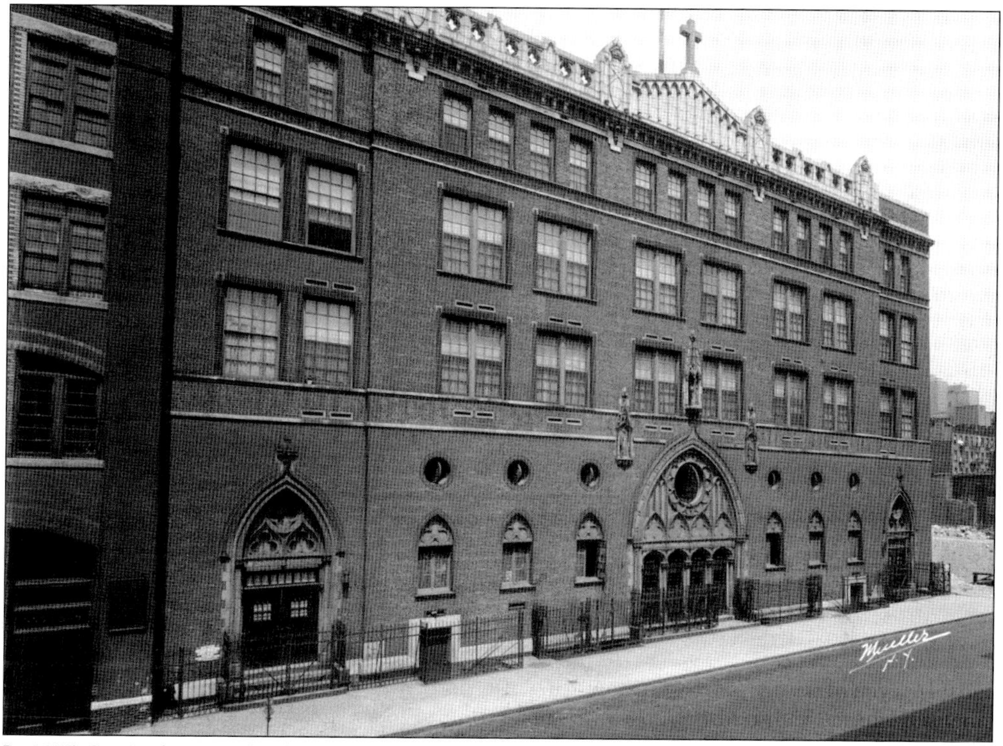

In 1935, St. Ambrose School and rectory in New York City were closed by the Archdiocese, and in return for the use of the buildings, the Carmelite Sisters paid the interest on the mortgage. Changes were made to the physical plant, and on November 21, 1935, the school became Mount Carmel Home, pictured here. It closed in 1981. This undated photograph was taken by Mueller Photography.

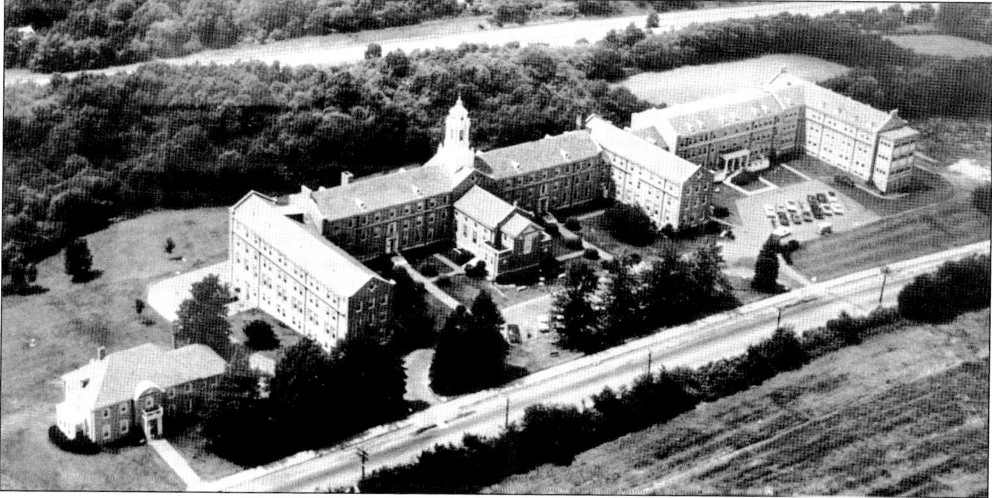

Catholic Memorial Home was built by the Diocese of Fall River, Massachusetts, in 1939, and Bishop James E. Cassidy chose the Carmelite Sisters for the Aged and Infirm to administer the facility. It originally accommodated 100 residents. In 1949, a new wing was added to bring the capacity up to 180, and in 1957, another wing was built that brought the total number of residents up to 300. For 64 years, the Carmelite Sisters cared for the elderly and sick at this facility, but in 2003, it was no longer possible to staff the home with sisters and they withdrew.

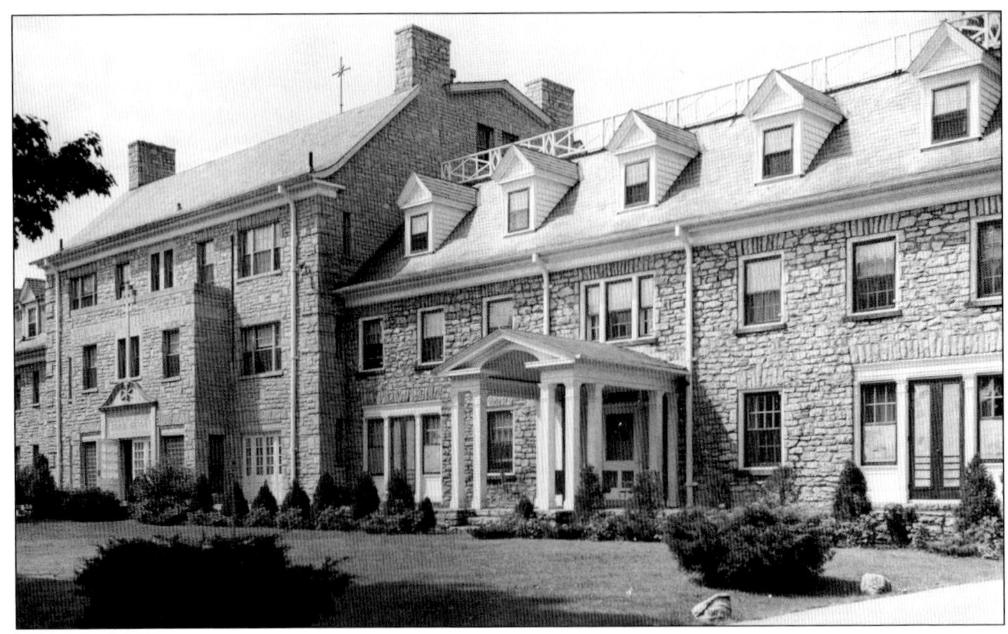

In 1946, Bishop Michael Ready of the Diocese of Columbus, Ohio, purchased a limestone mansion that formerly belonged to Samuel Prescott Bush, grandfather of George H.W. Bush and great-grandfather of George W. Bush and gave it to the Carmelite Sisters. The main building, called St. Raphael's Home, was used as a residence for the elderly, and a converted garage became a convent for the sisters. By 1949, a new wing was added to bring the home's capacity up to 85.

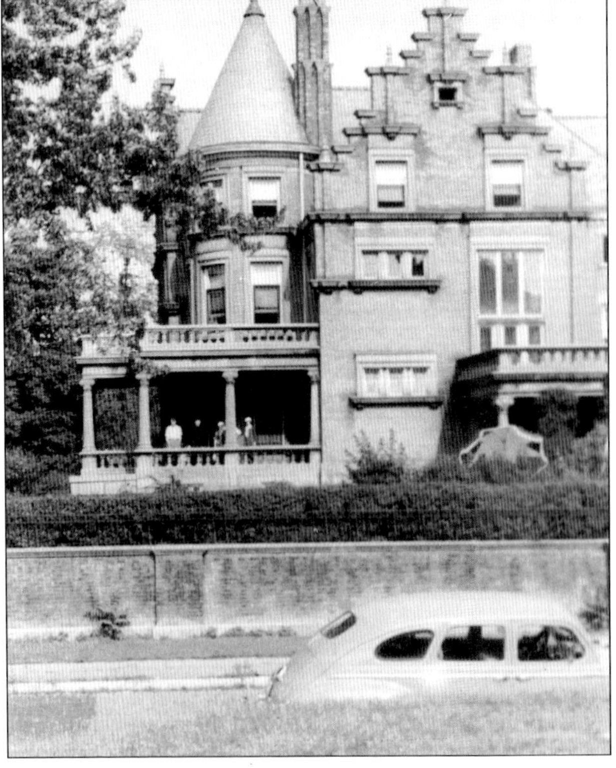

By 1948, St. Raphael's was filled to capacity. Bishop Ready bought an old Victorian mansion that had been operated by the Franciscan sisters as a home for working girls. He then gave the home to Mother Angeline so that the building could be renovated to care for the applicants on the waiting list for St. Raphael's Home. This facility was called St. Rita's Home and opened in 1949. It was expanded twice, but both St. Raphael's Home and St. Rita's Home could no longer be brought up to building codes, so the homes were combined in 2005 into a new facility in Columbus called Mother Angeline McCrory Manor.

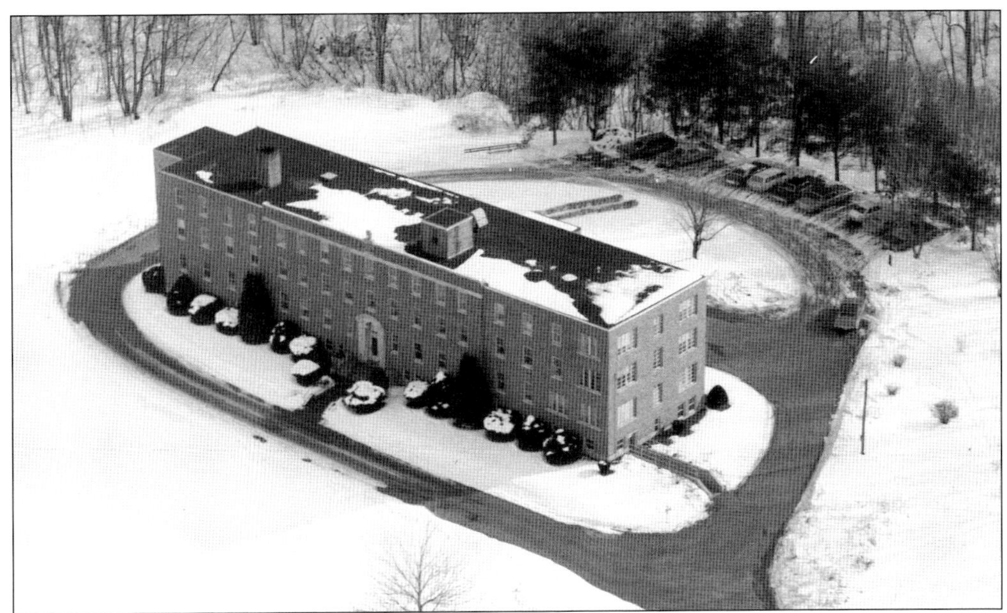

The first Mount Carmel Home in New Hampshire was opened by New Hampshire Catholic Charities in 1949 to care for 50 residents, and was one of three homes the Carmelite Sisters administered in New Hampshire. In 1969, a new facility was opened to welcome 125 residents and given the same name as the original one. The original home then became St. Teresa's Manor.

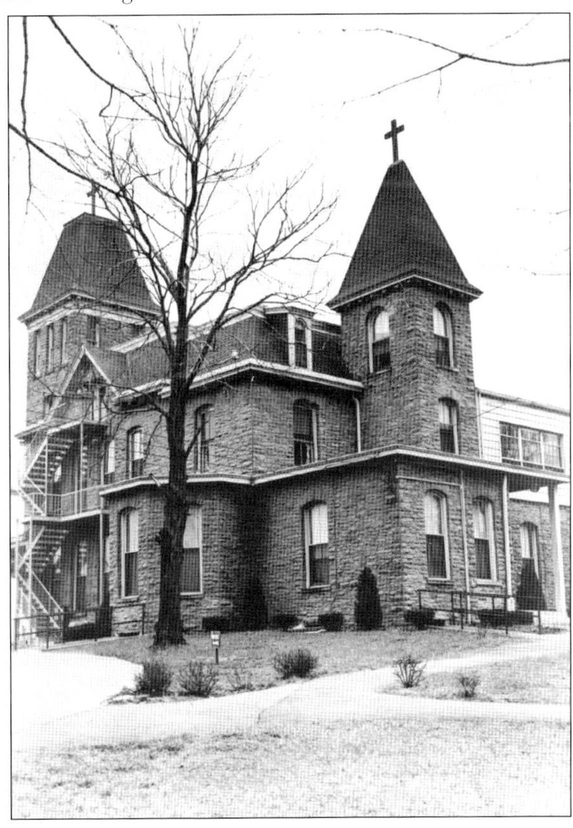

In 1949, Bishop William T. Molloy invited Mother Angeline and the Carmelite Sisters to open a nursing home in the Diocese of Covington, Kentucky. The original house bought by the bishop is pictured here. It housed 35 residents, but quickly became too small for the demand. Over the years, Carmel Manor was expanded with new additions, including a section for retired priests. It now welcomes 95 skilled residents and has a small personal care unit. Plans are being formulated to add more independent living and personal care units.

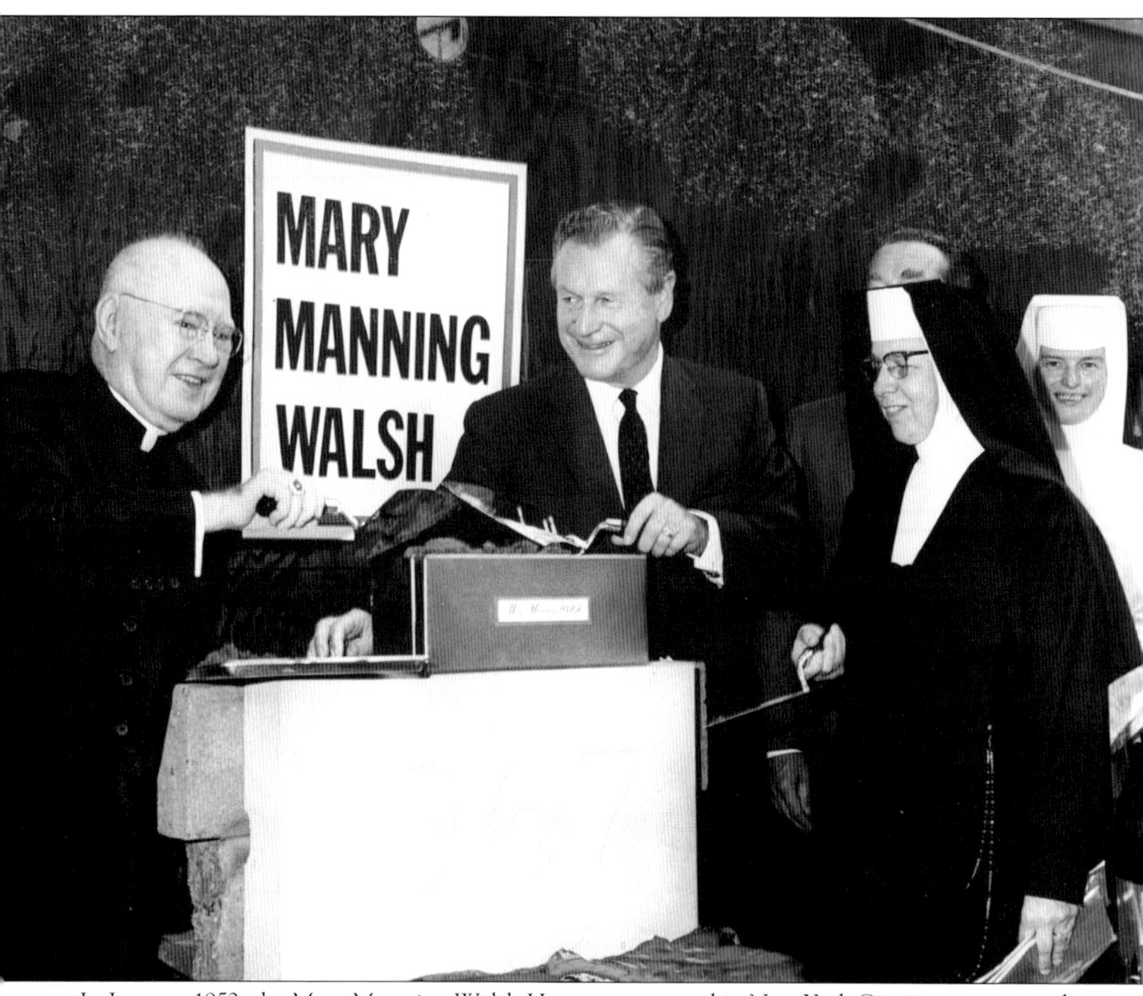

In January 1952, the Mary Manning Walsh Home was opened in New York City in a repurposed building. By 1969, it became impossible to remodel the home according to new building codes and the medical needs of the residents. A new building was erected on a different site in New York City. From left to right, Cardinal Spellman, Gov. Nelson Rockefeller, and Mother Aloysius are laying the cornerstone for the new 16-story facility, which would house 362 residents.

Over the years, several fundraisers were held to help the Carmelite Sisters provide care for the residents at Mary Manning Walsh Home. In this photograph, Mother Aloysius, administrator at the time, can be seen with Princess Grace of Monaco, who graciously chaired one of the fundraisers.

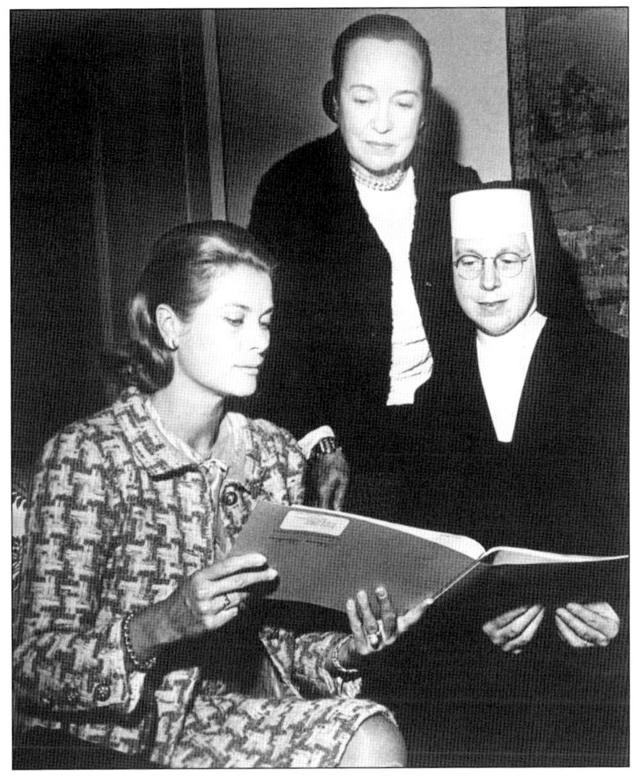

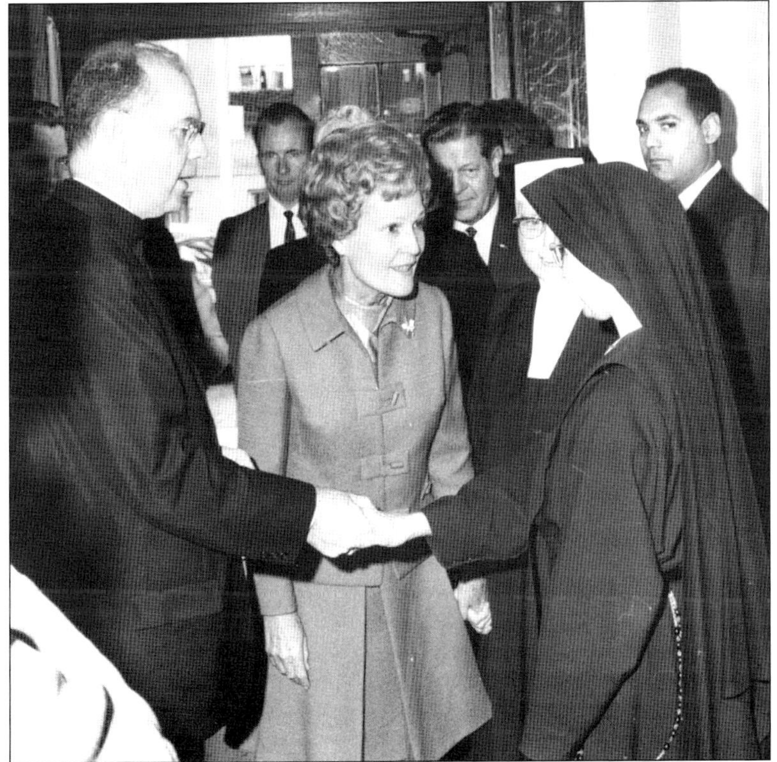

Terence Cardinal Cooke was a large supporter of Mary Manning Walsh Home. Here, he is presenting First Lady Pat Nixon to Mother Aloysius (left) and Mother Bernadette, who both served many years as administrators of the facility.

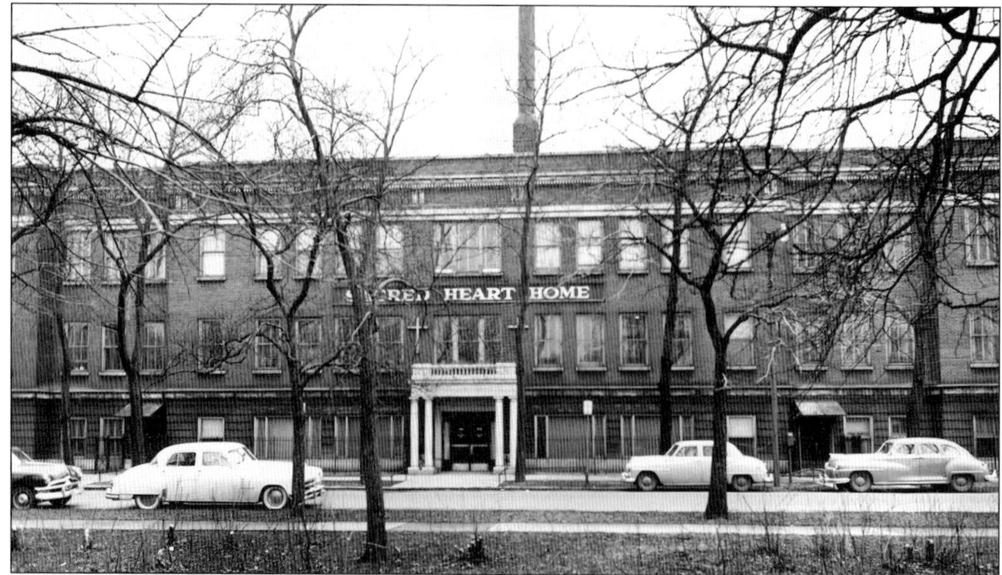

Sacred Heart Home in Chicago was founded by the Carmelite Sisters on June 22, 1950, in a former Jewish orphanage and converted into a nursing home with a capacity of 200 residents. The sisters had previously taken over the care of St. Mary's Day Nursery and were known for their loving care in the archdiocese. The facility was closed in 1972.

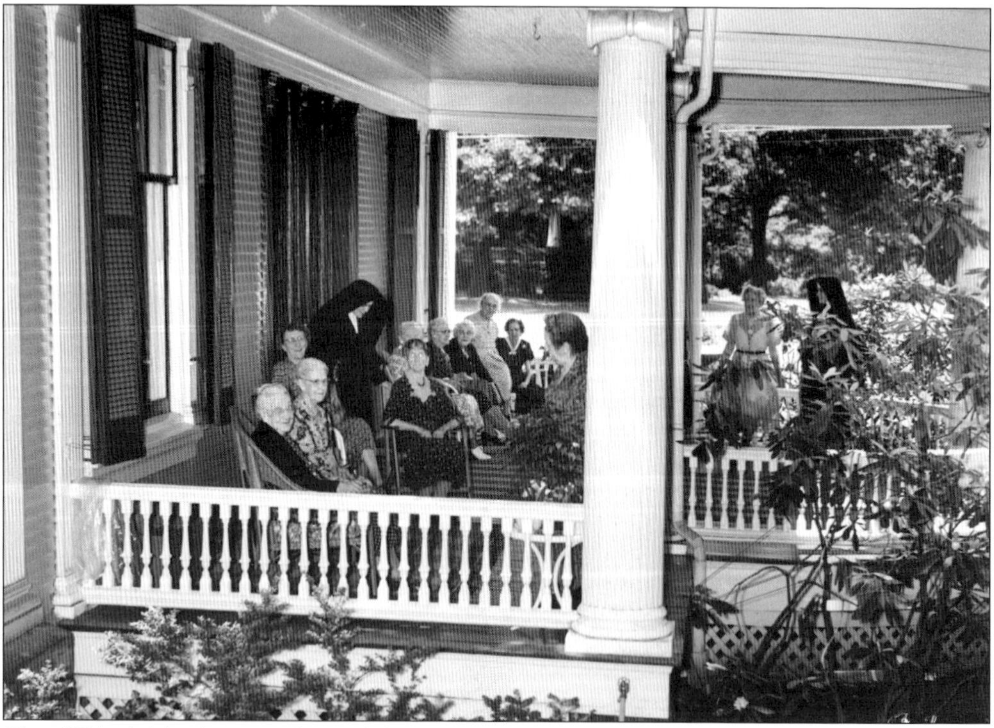

Clara Welty left her home to the Archdiocese of Wheeling, West Virginia, and Archbishop Thomas J. McDonnell asked the Carmelite Sisters to operate the Welty Home, which accommodated only 16 residents. When a larger home was unable to be built, the sisters withdrew and returned to the motherhouse in 1961.

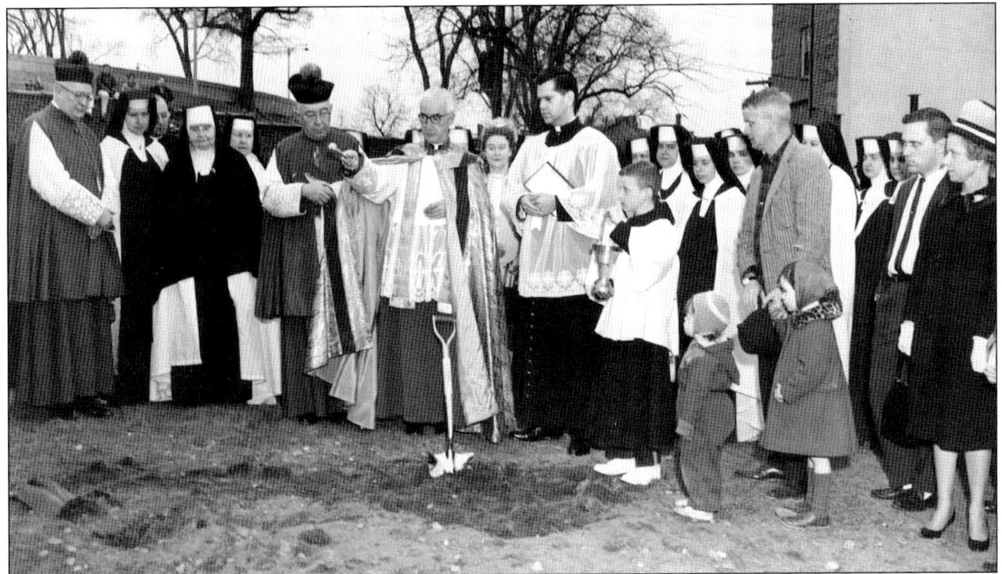

In 1953, Cardinal Cushing invited Mother Angeline to send sisters to South Boston to take over the facilities of the historic Carney Hospital. The hospital was transformed into Marian Manor Nursing Home and had a capacity to serve 150. By 1962, the waiting list was so long that a building program was undertaken to increase the capacity to 250, and in 1974, another wing of 120 beds was added. This is the ground-breaking ceremony for one of the construction projects.

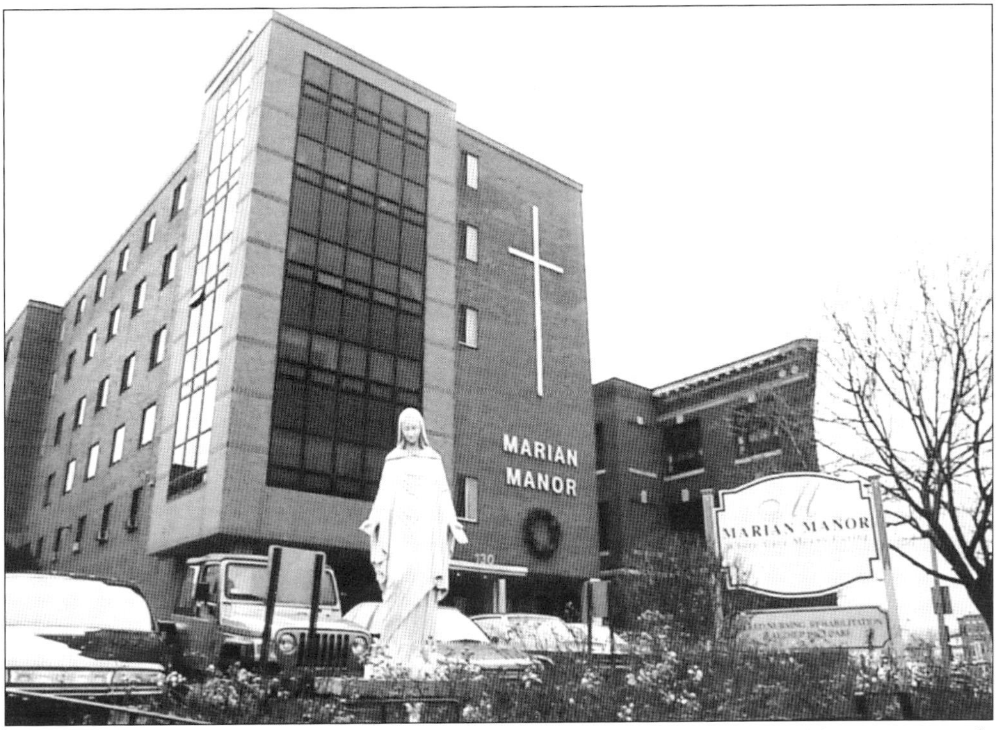

The facility today is a collection of four buildings attached to one another as additions were made over the years. At the time of this publication, the Carmelite Sisters are exploring options for a new state-of-the-art facility to provide for the needs of their residents.

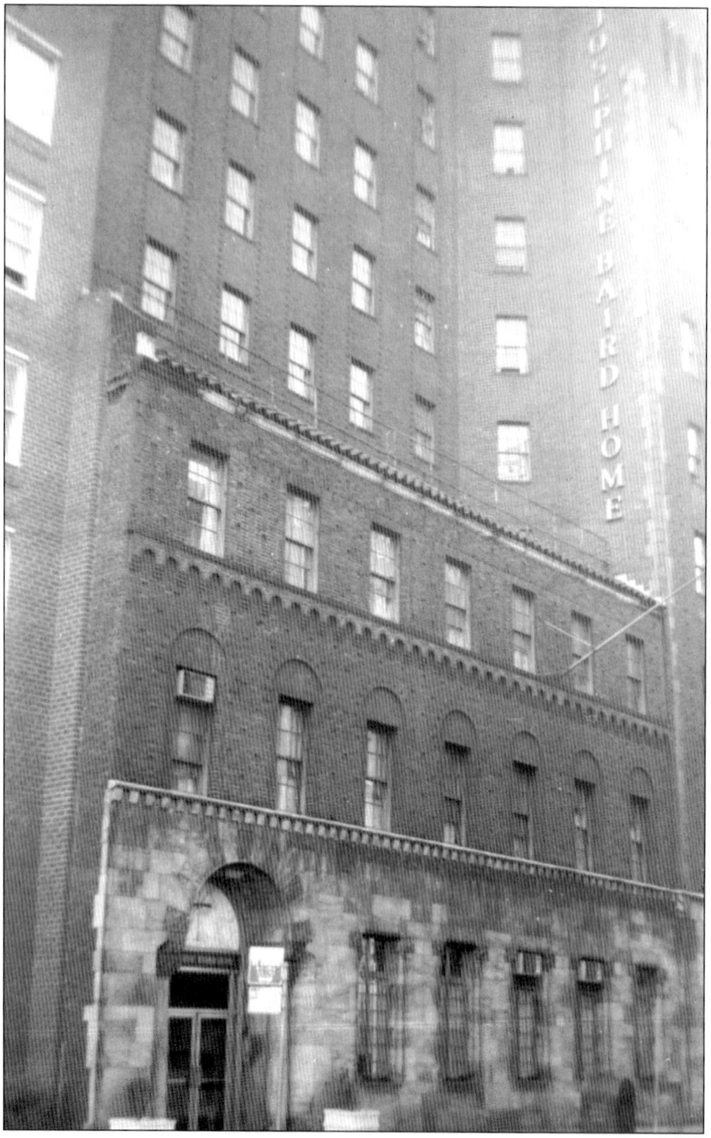

Josephine Baird Home in New York City was founded in February 1955 after Francis Cardinal Spellman bought the property, which had been known as Shelton College, a training seminary conducted by the National Bible Society. It was converted into a nursing home to accommodate 179 residents. The facility was closed in 1972 when it could no longer be brought up to building codes.

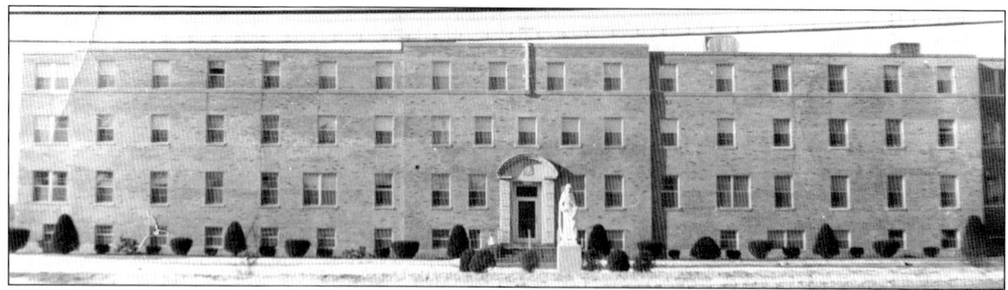

In 1958, Bishop Matthew F. Brady blessed and dedicated St. Ann Home in Dover, New Hampshire. It had a capacity of 52 residents, and provided skilled nursing care, medical services, rehabilitation services, dental, podiatry, occupational and recreational therapy, and pastoral care for all denominations.

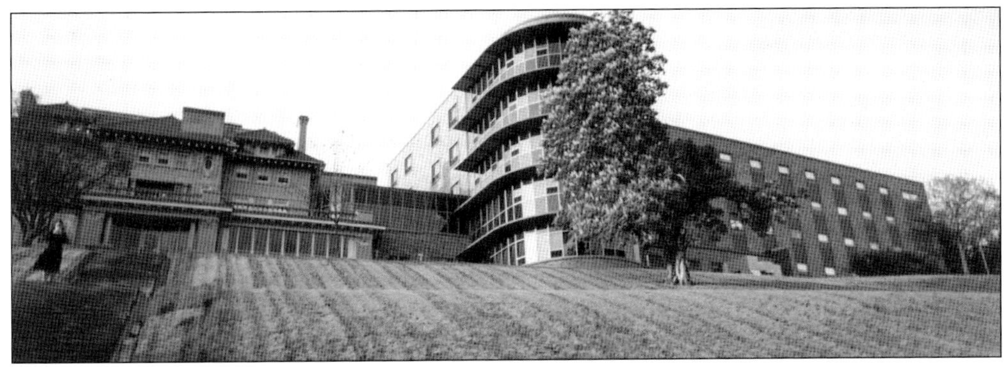

In 1954, Bishop Ralph L. Hayes received the donation of the Kahl family home on six acres. It was to become a nursing home administered by the Carmelite Sisters along with a memorial to the family. Within a few years, an addition was needed due to the demand for admission. The original Kahl Home for the Aged can be seen here to the left of the new addition, which was built in 1963 and brought the capacity to 150.

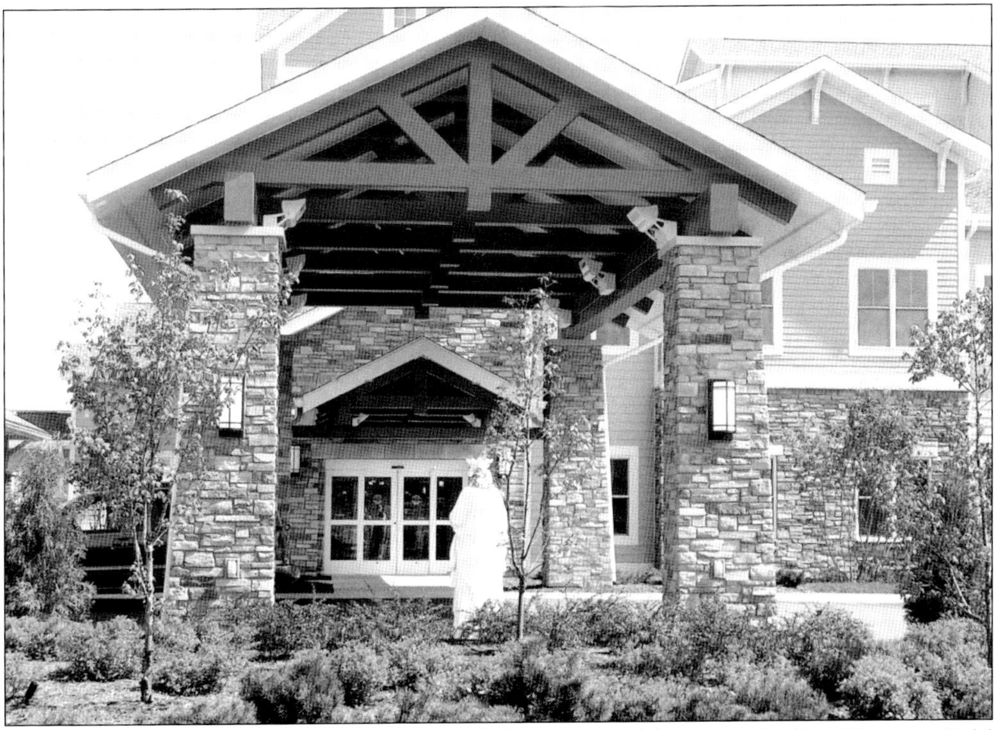

Increasing demand and aging infrastructure led to the need for a new facility. The new Kahl Home for the Aged (pictured) was opened in 2012, and skilled care is provided for 135 residents. Sufficient land was purchased to add independent living and assisted living at a later date.

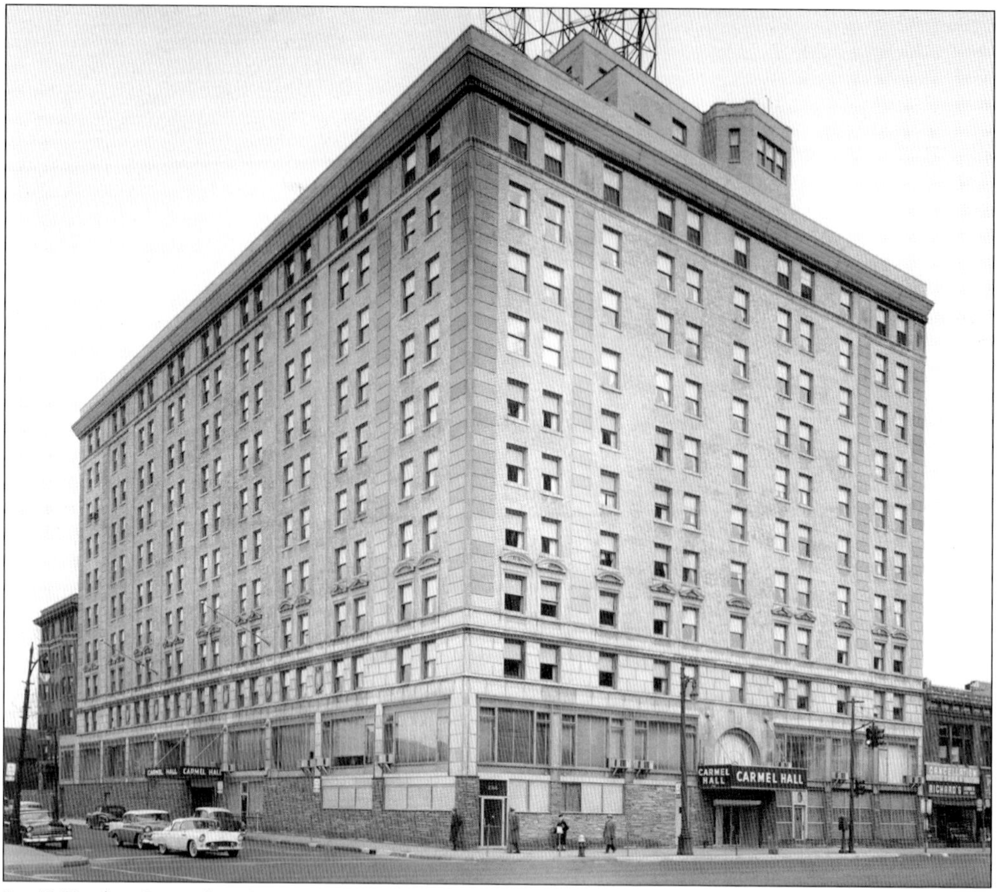

In 1955, the Carmelite Sisters transformed the Detroiter Hotel into Carmel Hall and provided care for 500 residents in Detroit, Michigan. The sisters withdrew in 1979.

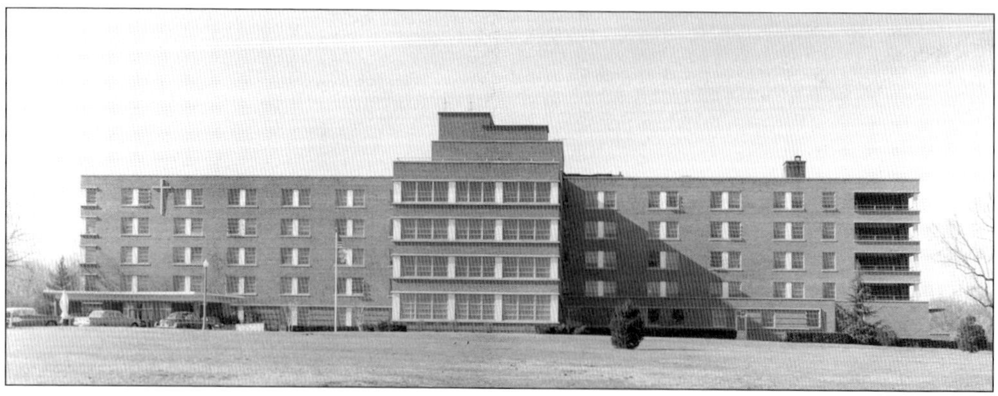

In 1949, Mother Angeline was invited to take over two homes in the Georgetown area of Washington, DC: the Catholic Home for Aged Ladies and the St. Margaret Mary House next door. Renovations were soon needed for those homes, but zoning regulations did not permit a new, larger facility. A new home, pictured here and named Carroll Manor, was then built in Prince George's County, Maryland, just outside Washington. It not only accommodated residents from the two Georgetown facilities but also had room for 250 residents in all. The sisters withdrew in 1991.

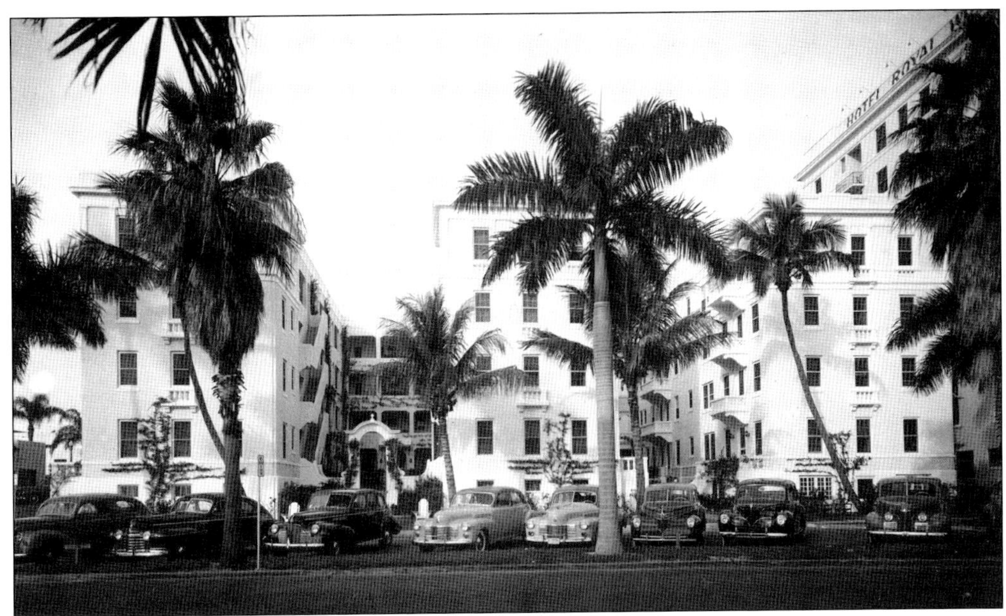

The Lake Court Hotel in West Palm Beach, Florida, was acquired by the sisters and converted into Lourdes Residence. Dedicated in February 1961, it became inadequate for the care of the elderly and was closed in 1975. Mrs. John T. McKeen donated $1 million toward the cost of rebuilding a nursing home on the same site. The new facility, named the Lourdes-Noreen McKeen Residence, was dedicated in December 1980.

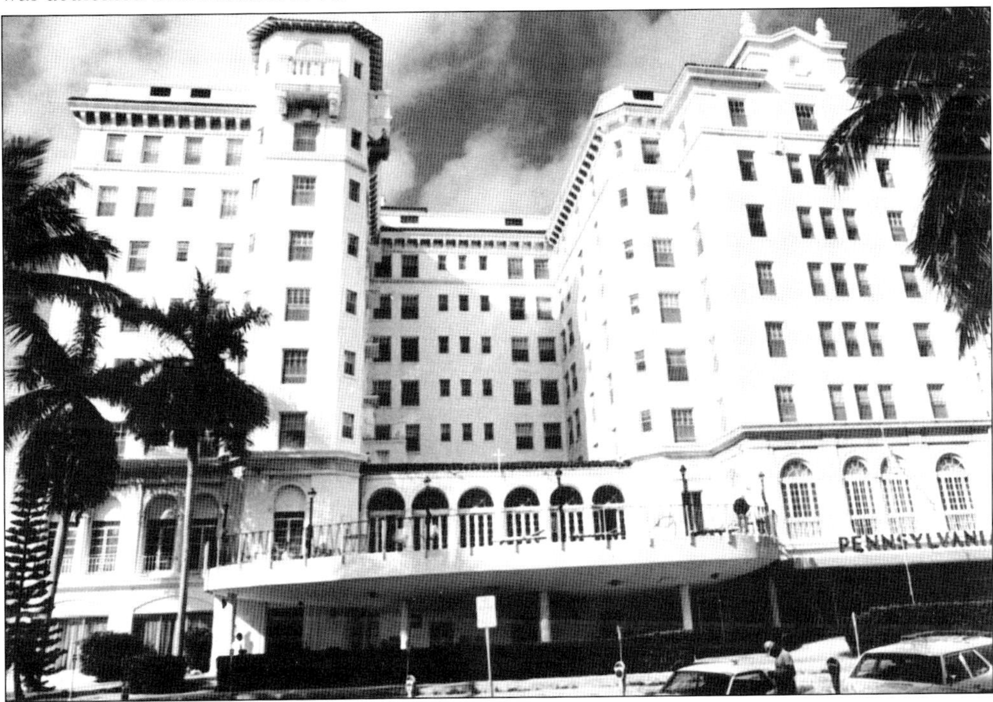

Next door to Lourdes Residence stood the 250-room Pennsylvania Hotel, which the Carmelite Sisters administered as the first retirement hotel under Catholic auspices in the Diocese of Miami. It welcomed seasonal as well as year-round residents.

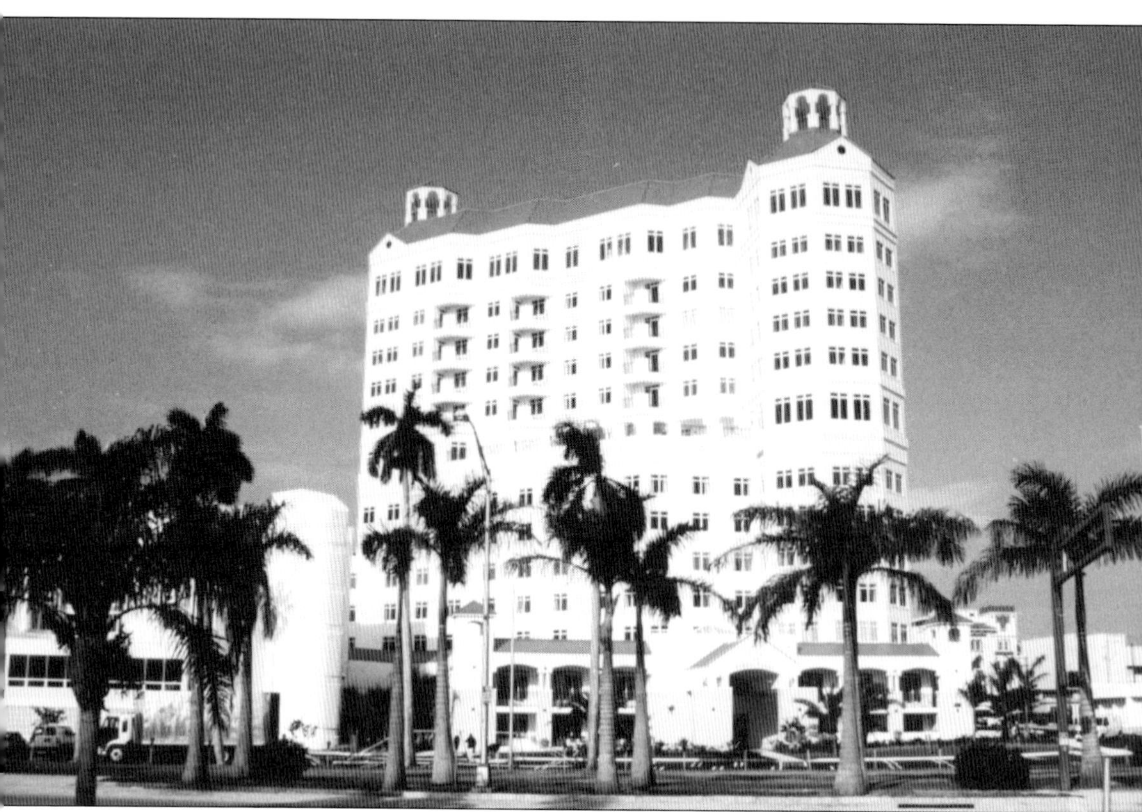

The Pennsylvania Hotel was imploded in 1995 and the McKeen Towers building was constructed on the site of the old hotel. It offers both assisted living and independent living apartments and stands side by side with the nursing facility. The total on-site capacity of all levels of care is 251.

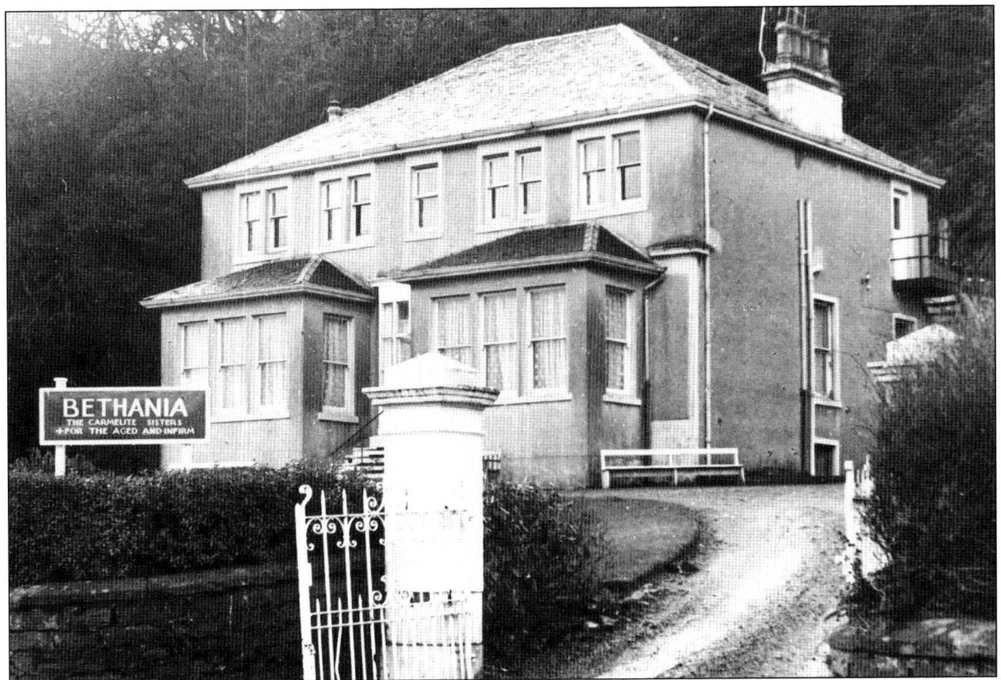

This facility in Dunoon, Scotland, was named Bethania and had been managed by a small group of four sisters whose foundress had died. In 1964, the Bishop of Argyll, Stephen McGill, asked Mother Angeline to take over the operation of the facility.

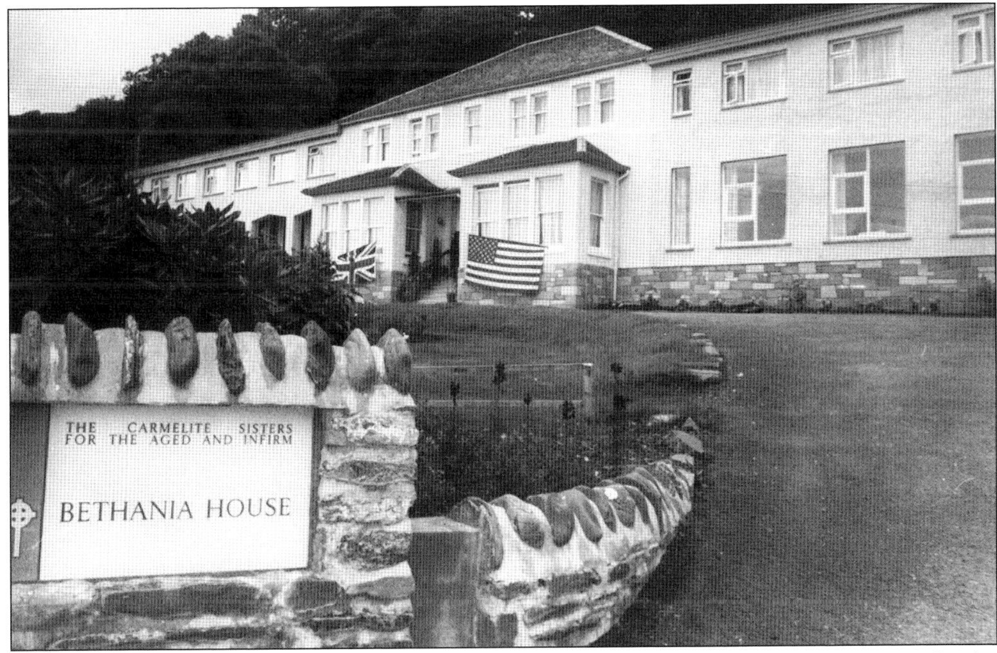

Mother Angeline planned an addition because the house was too small to properly care for the elderly. This addition increased the capacity to 40 residents. The Carmelite Sisters withdrew in 1976 because they were needed back in the United States. Bethania was then taken over by a social service agency in Glasgow.

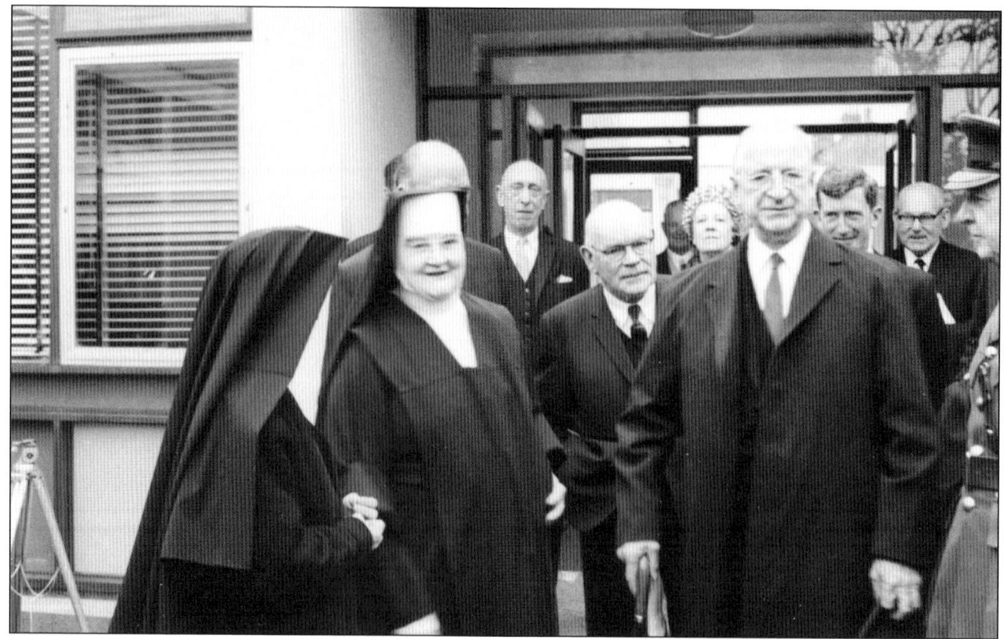

Archbishop John C. McQuaid, hearing of the Carmelite Sisters' care for the elderly in the United States, invited Mother Angeline to open a home in Dublin, Ireland. In 1961, land, including Bullock Castle, was purchased in Dalkey, just south of Dublin. This photograph taken in 1965 shows Ireland's president Eamon de Valera with Mother Angeline and other dignitaries at the Mass of dedication of the new facility called Our Lady's Manor.

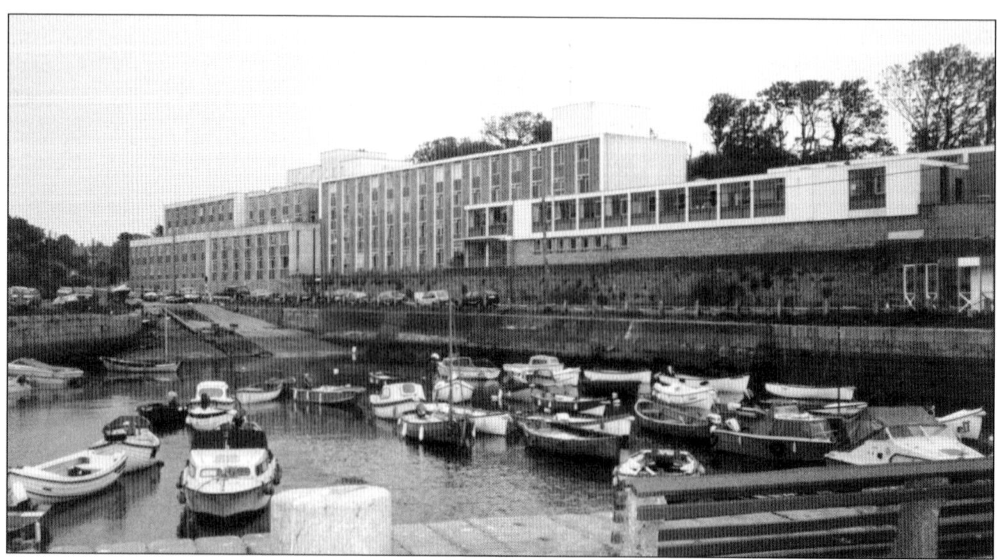

Our Lady's Manor is located right on the Irish Sea, as can be seen in this photograph. The original facility's size was augmented by additional buildings, bringing the capacity to 175 residents.

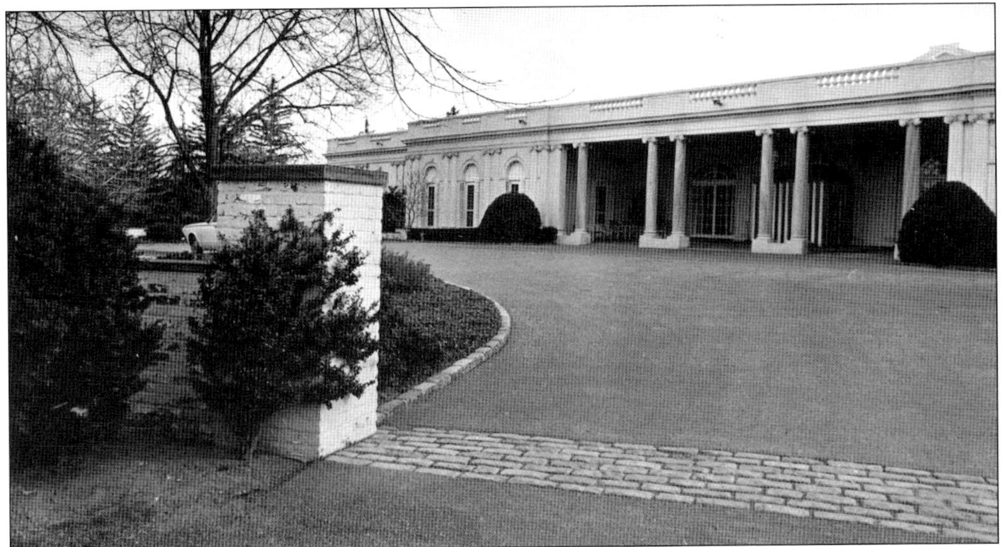

In 1964, Brooke Astor donated her home and some adjoining land to the Archdiocese of New York, and Cardinal Spellman invited the Carmelite Sisters to administer it as a retirement home for 20 residents. The home, called Ferncliff, pictured here, was actually the tennis house that was part of the original William Astor mansion built in 1855 and demolished in 1945.

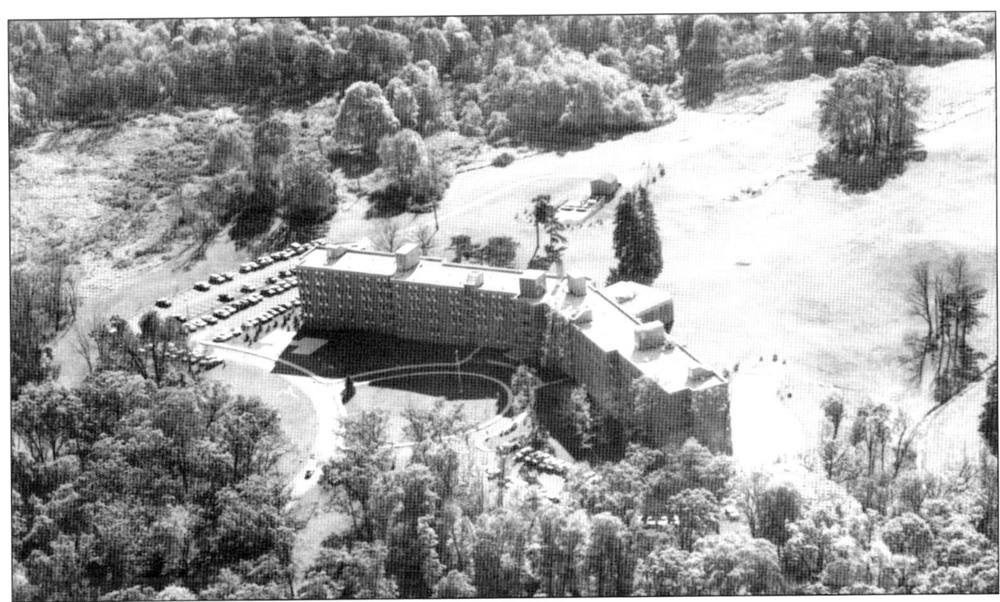

Cardinal Spellman immediately set about finding financing for a much larger facility. In October 1972, his successor, Archbishop Terrence Cooke, helped lay the cornerstone of the new Ferncliff nursing home pictured here. It was built to provide nursing care to 320 elderly residents under the auspices of the archdiocese and the supervision of the Carmelite Sisters. The sisters withdrew in 2009.

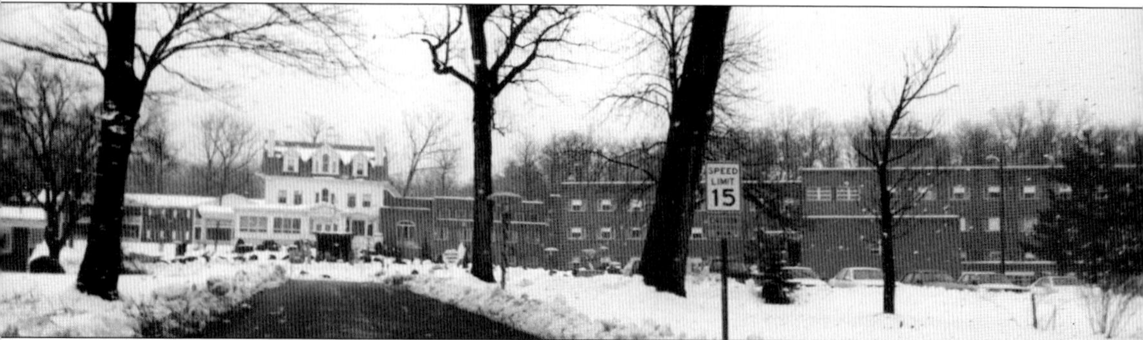

Garvey Manor, located in Hollidaysburg, Pennsylvania, opened its doors in April 1965 and had a capacity of 154 residents. It is co-sponsored by the Diocese of Altoona-Johnstown and the Carmelite Sisters. An addition was constructed in 1980 to add two dining rooms and storage space. In the late 1990s, the board determined that a new facility of 132 beds with more private rooms was needed, as well as a component of 54 assisted living units.

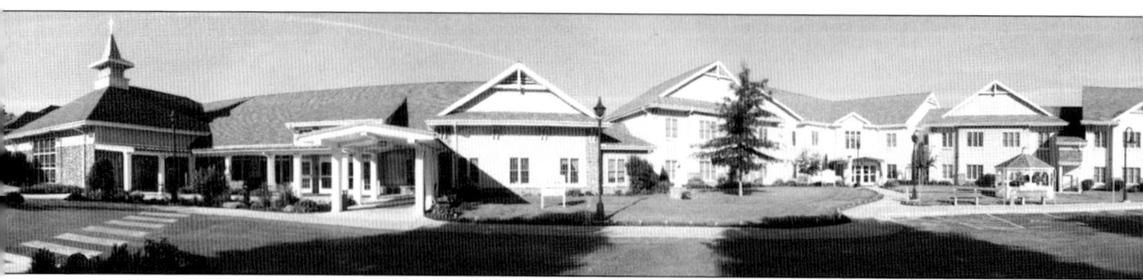

The new Garvey Manor, opened on another part of the site in 2003, is pictured here and provides a continuum of care from independent to skilled. The old facility was demolished and expansion of independent units is planned for the future.

In 1964, the Carmelite Sisters purchased the Louis Joliet Hotel in Joliet, Illinois, with the firm intention of converting it into a residence for the aged. It was renamed the St. Patrick Retirement Hotel and dedicated in June 1965. It had a capacity of 197 and operated until 1989, when a new facility was built.

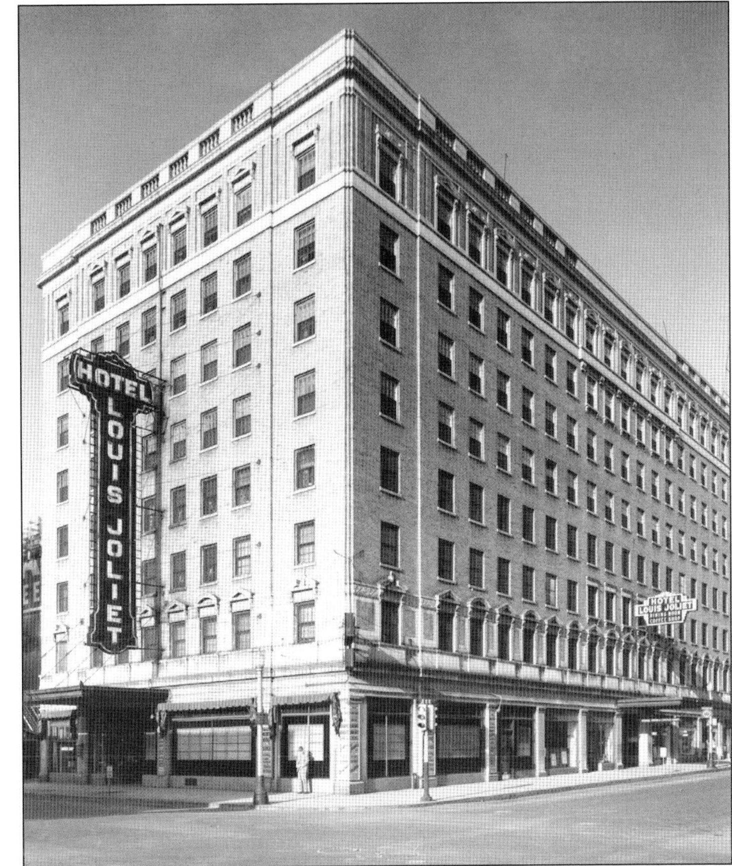

The new St. Patrick's Residence opened in Naperville, Illinois, in 1989. It has a capacity of 194 residents.

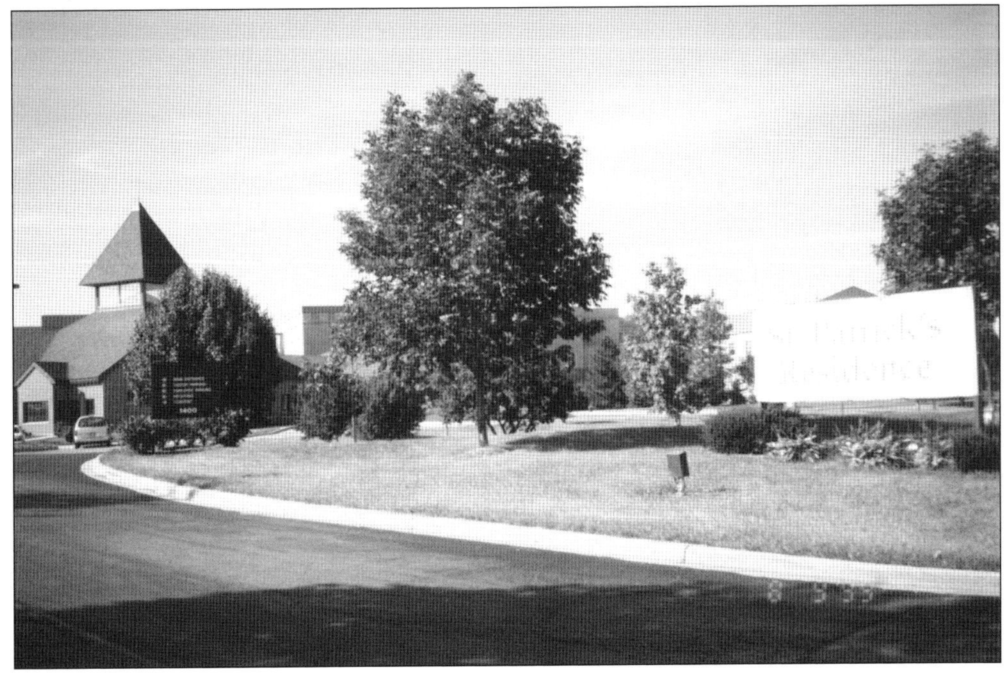

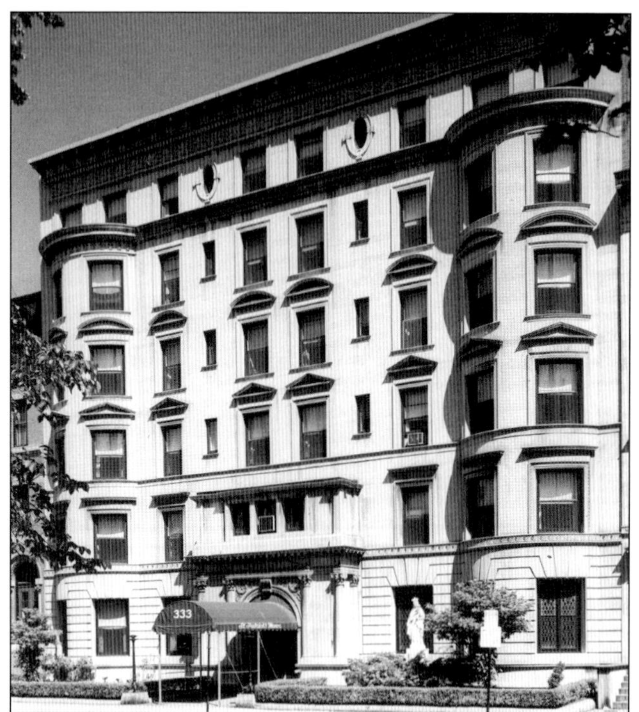

In 1953, Richard Cardinal Cushing of the Archdiocese of Boston purchased the Lafayette Hotel in Boston and the Carmelite Sisters renovated it and renamed it St. Patrick's Manor. It operated for 11 years at this location before it became necessary to move due to the constant need for major repairs and maintenance.

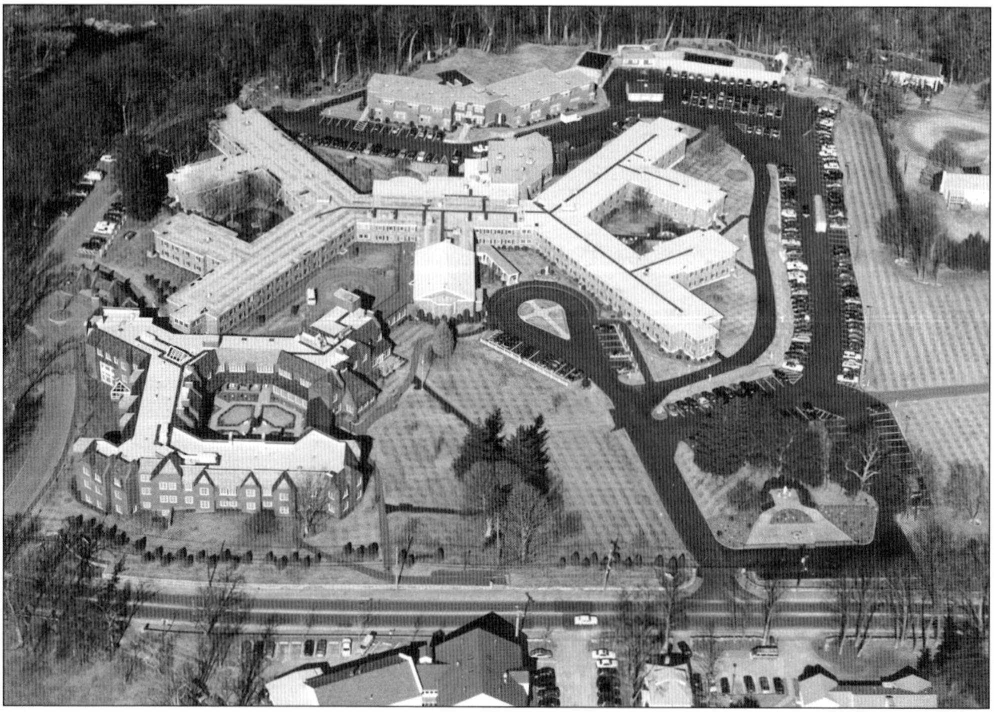

In 1964, Cardinal Cushing gave the sisters property in Framingham, Massachusetts, and they constructed a new St. Patrick's Manor. The new home pictured here opened in 1970. (At lower left is Carmel Terrace, an assisted-living facility built by the Carmelite Sisters in 1995). St. Patrick's Manor presently accommodates 292 residents.

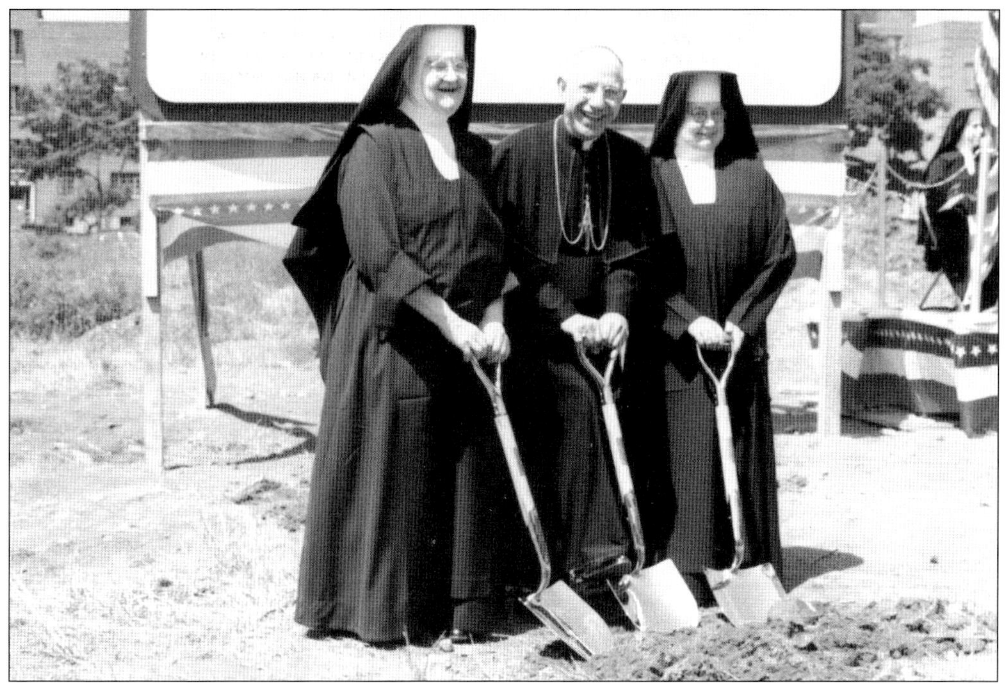

From left to right, Mother Angeline, Bishop Francis J. Mugavero, and Mother M. Ignatius Loyola are participating in the ground-breaking ceremony for the construction of the 11-story Ozanam Hall in Bayside, Queens, New York. The building opened in November 1971 and has a capacity of 432 residents.

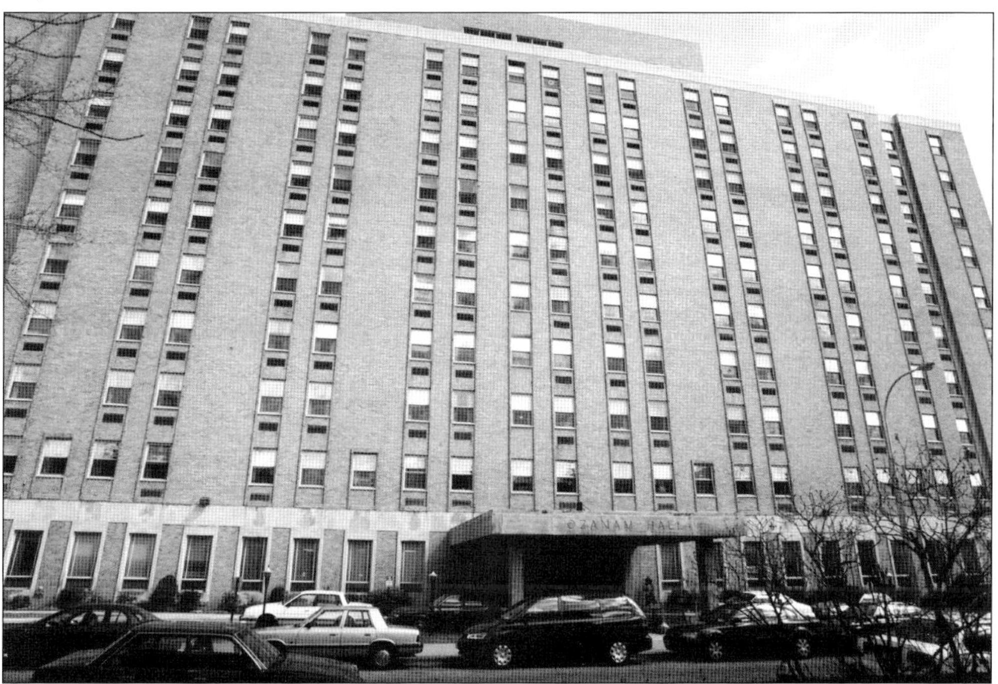

Ozanam Hall is co-sponsored by the Carmelite Sisters and the Diocese of Brooklyn. It was remodeled in 2011 and is administered by the Carmelite Sisters.

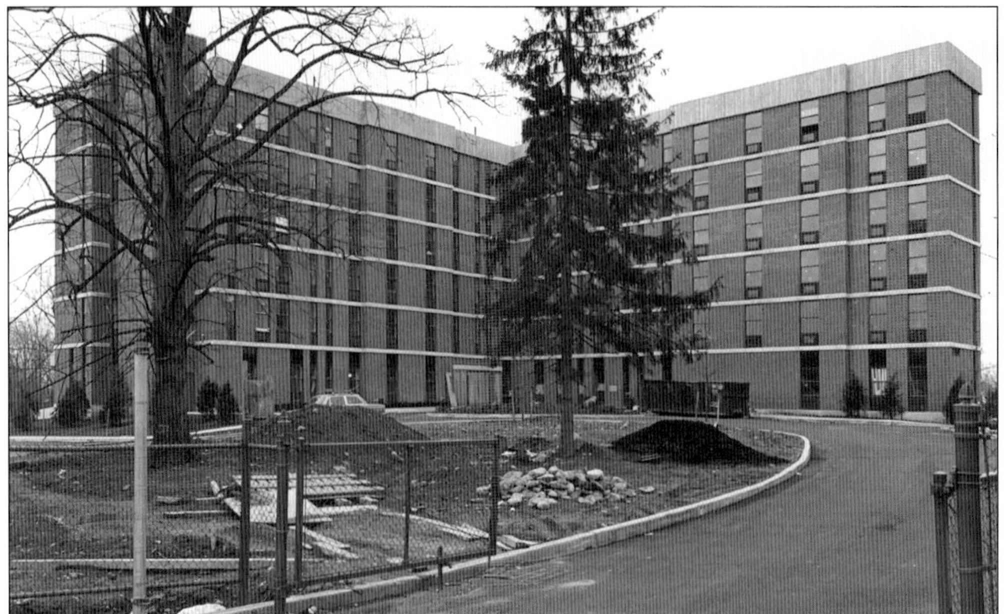

Carmel Richmond, located in Staten Island and sponsored by the Archdiocese of New York through ArchCare, is administered by the Carmelite Sisters. It opened in October 1974 and has a capacity of 300 residents. On the same site, ArchCare also offers a PACE program (Programs of All-Inclusive Care for the Elderly) for elderly persons who qualify for nursing care but prefer to remain in their own homes.

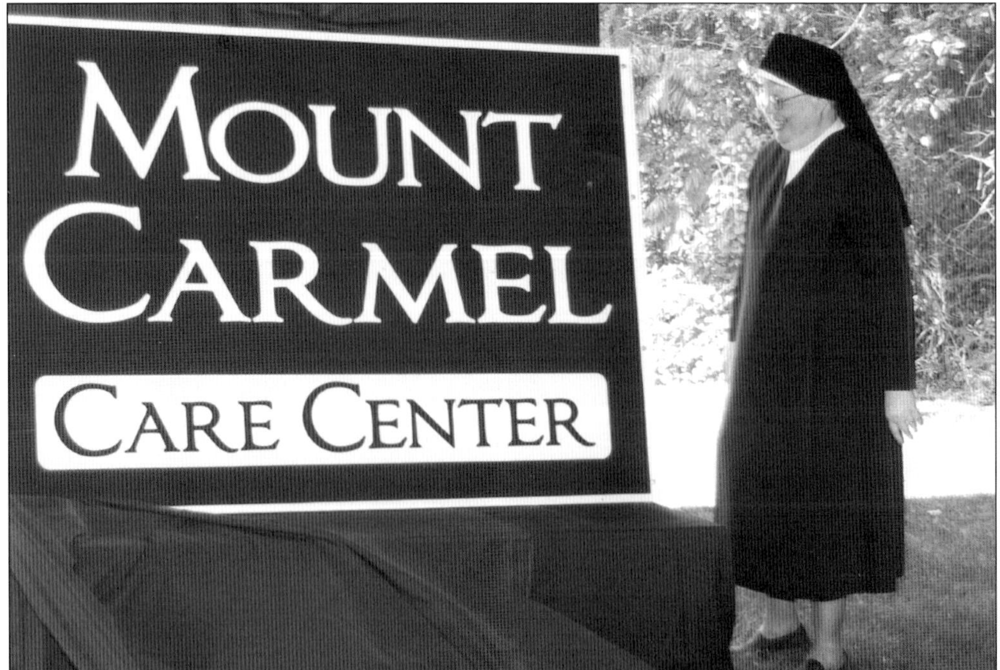

Mount Carmel Care Center, a 69-bed facility, was acquired by the Carmelite Sisters from the Sisters of Providence and is located in Lenox, Massachusetts. Here, Mother Mark Louis Anne unveils the new name of the facility at its rededication in 2013.

Three

THE SISTERS AT WORK

In the early days, the elderly who sought admission to the sisters' nursing homes were in generally good health and helped to do the cooking, small maintenance, and some gardening. In later years, those admitted for care were in poorer health and needed more specialized nursing care. In the 1950s, Mother Angeline began sending some sisters to school to become licensed nurses, lab technicians, social workers, dietitians, and therapists.

The sisters believe that care of the elderly should encompass all aspects of the person: their physical, social, psychological, spiritual, and emotional needs. As Mother Angeline said in her 1968 Easter letter to the sisters, "Our apostolate is not only to operate up-to-date homes for the aged. As religious, we bring Christ to every person in our care. Bringing Christ means giving people His compassion, His interest, His loving care—His warmth, morning, noon and night. It means inspiring the lay people who work with us to give the same type of loving care."

The photographs in this chapter show the sisters providing that loving care to their residents. It is important to note the changes in the veil; the first change was in 1960 and became necessary because the wider veil inhibited vision while driving. The new veil was then replaced by a more modern version in 1972.

Some photographs also show the sisters in white habits, which were an option for the sisters in the nursing homes; the white habit did not necessarily indicate that the sister was a nurse.

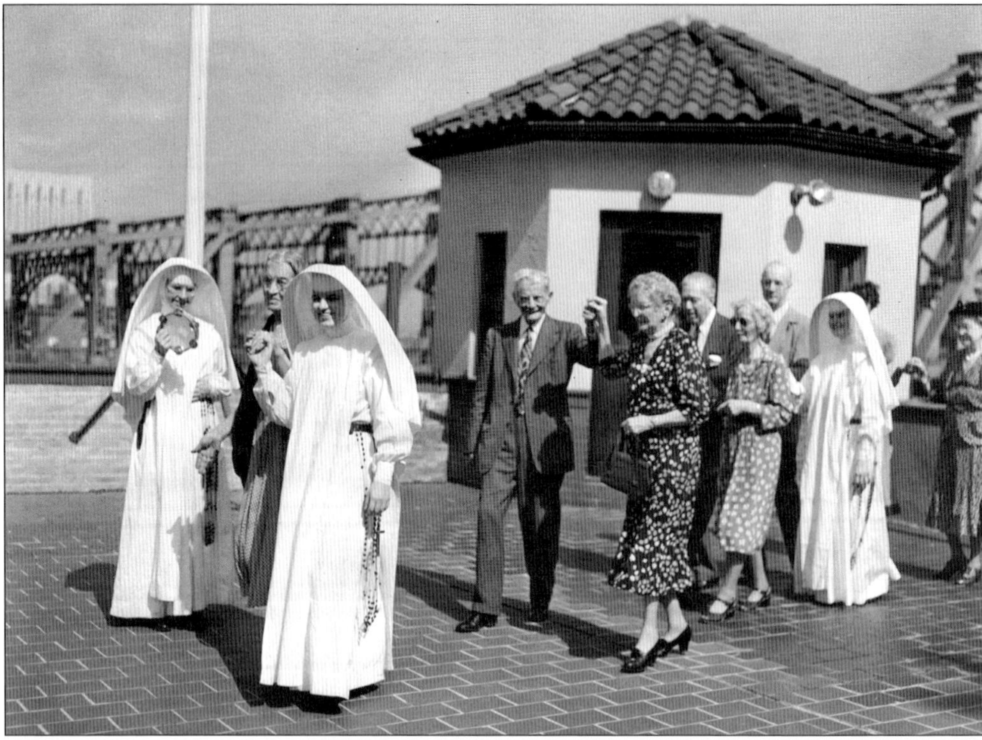

The sisters lead the residents in a dance on the rooftop of the old Mary Manning Walsh Home on Fifty-Ninth Street in New York City.

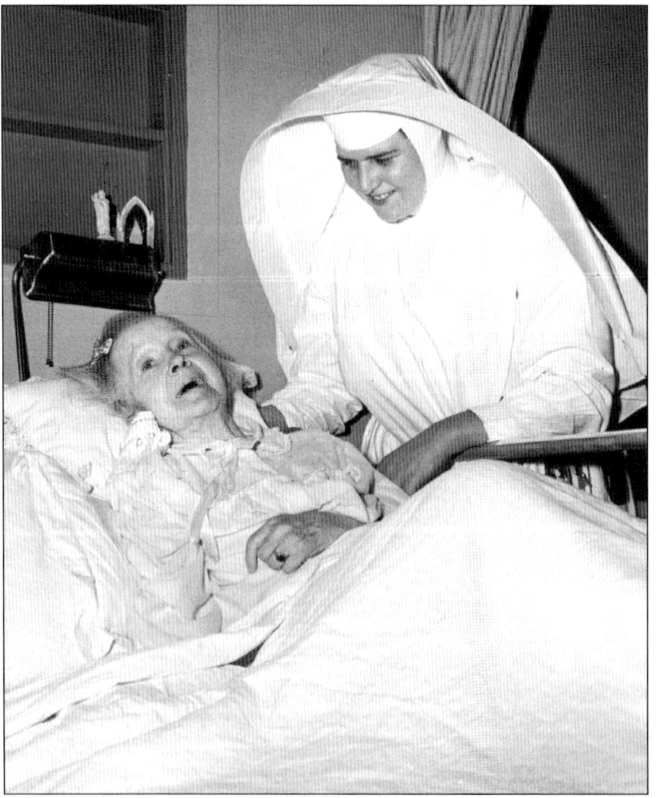

Sr. Daniel Marie is seen here ministering to a resident. Over the years, she always provided a loving, resident-centered approach to those under her care.

A sister nurse provides a treatment to one of her residents.

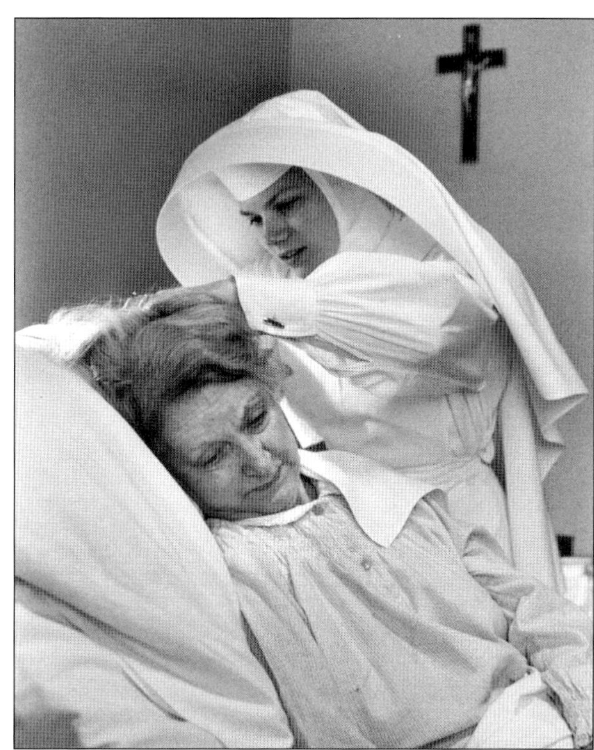

Postulant Sr. Julia Marie and Sr. Fidelis Regan cheer up a resident confined to bed.

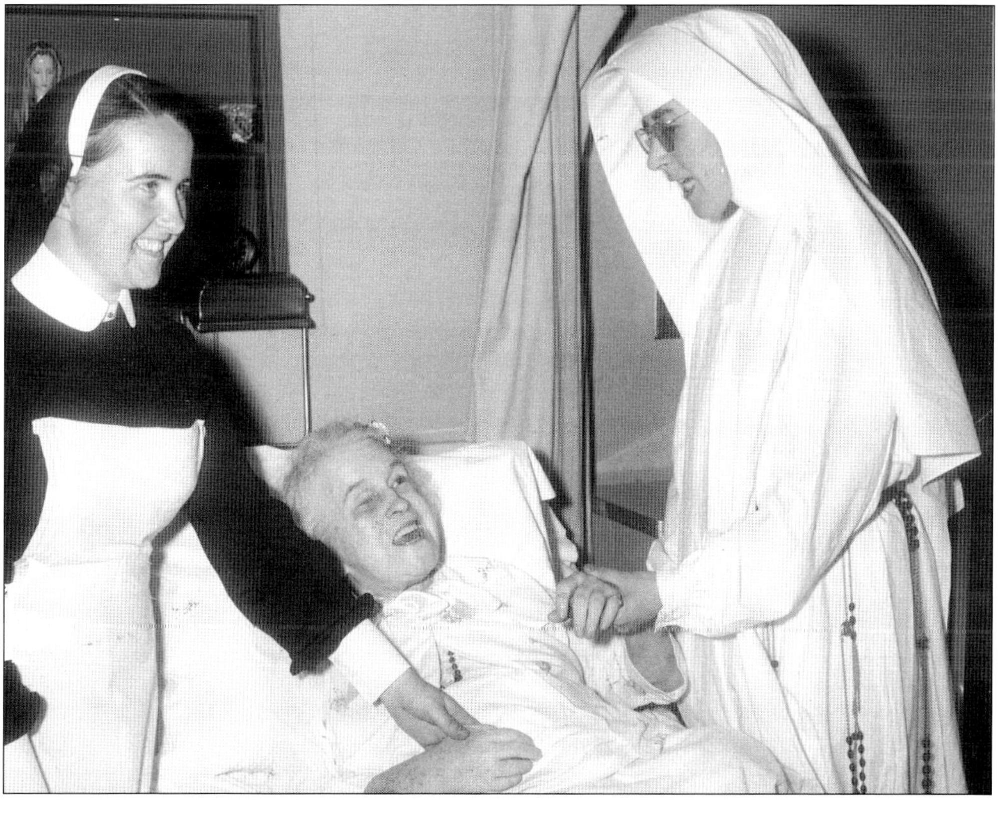

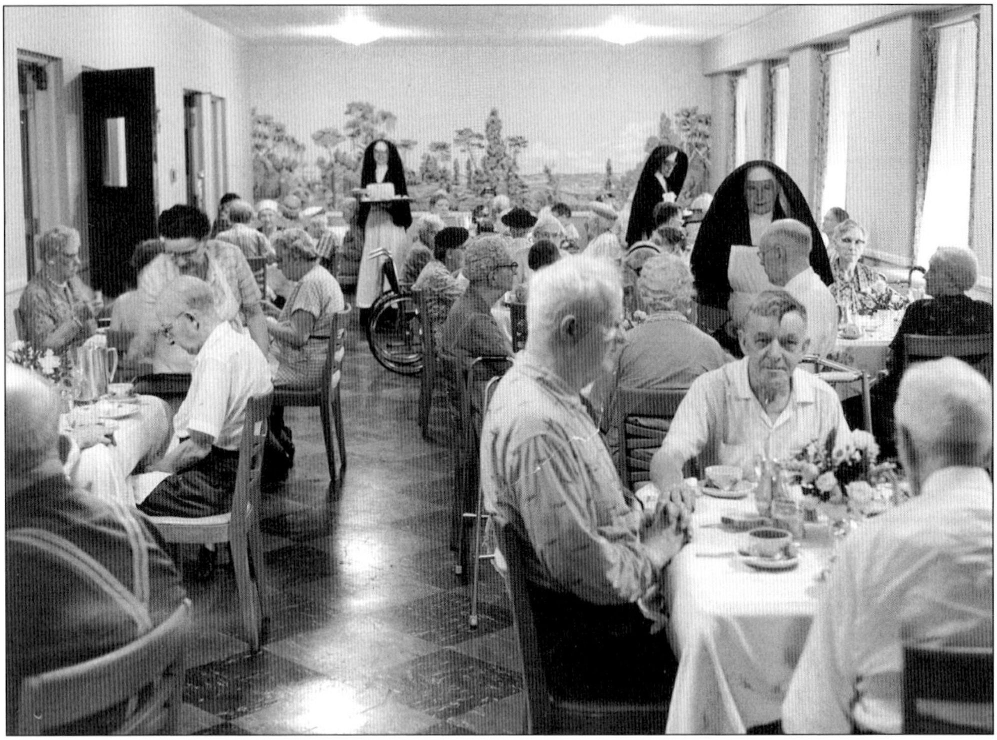

Three sisters are serving residents their meals in this photograph. The tables are set with fine china, and flowers adorn every table.

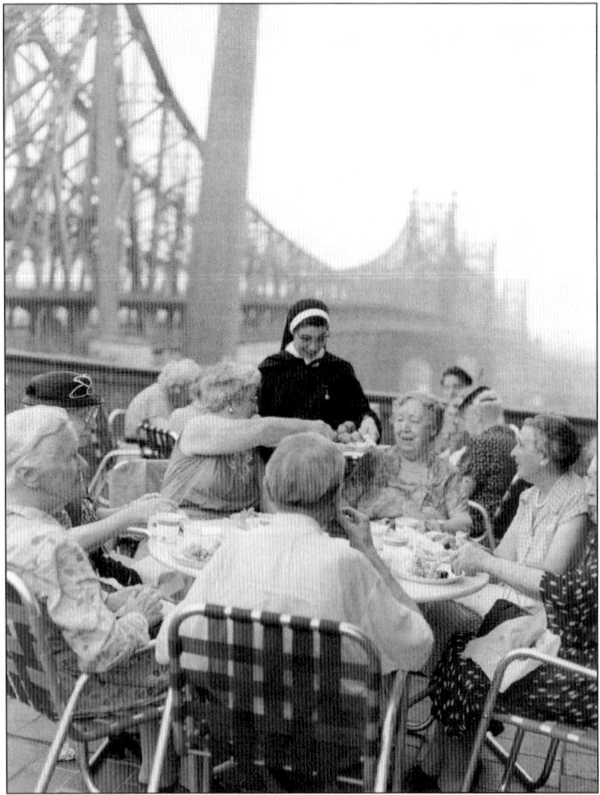

A postulant is serving residents on the rooftop of the old Mary Manning Walsh Home, with the Fifty-Ninth Street Bridge in the background.

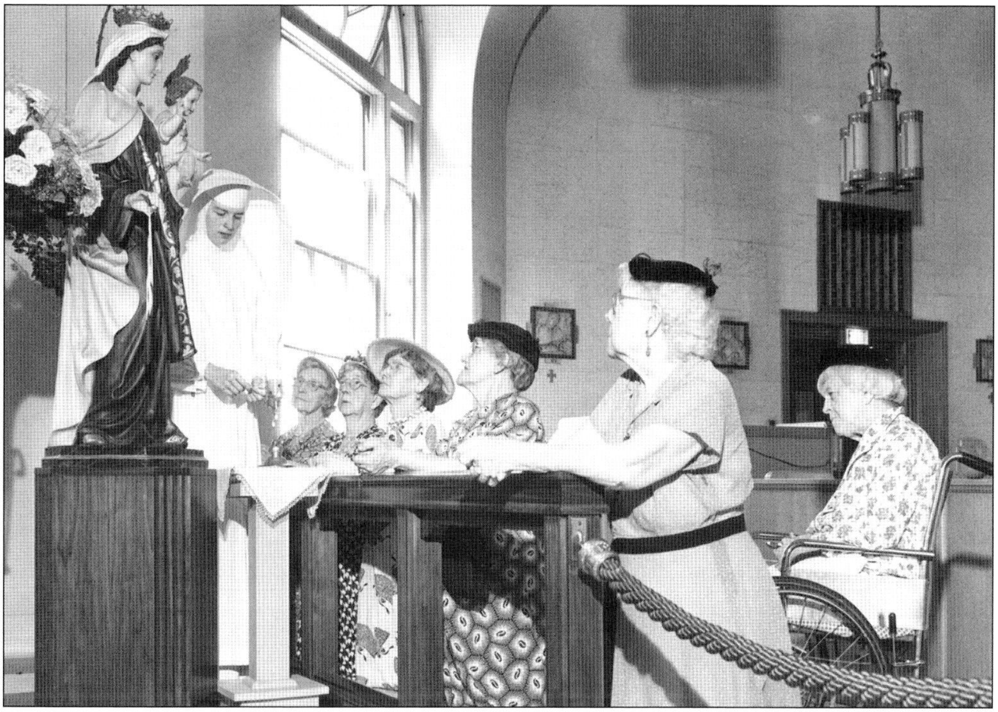

Standing beside a statue of Our Lady of Mount Carmel, a young sister leads residents in the rosary.

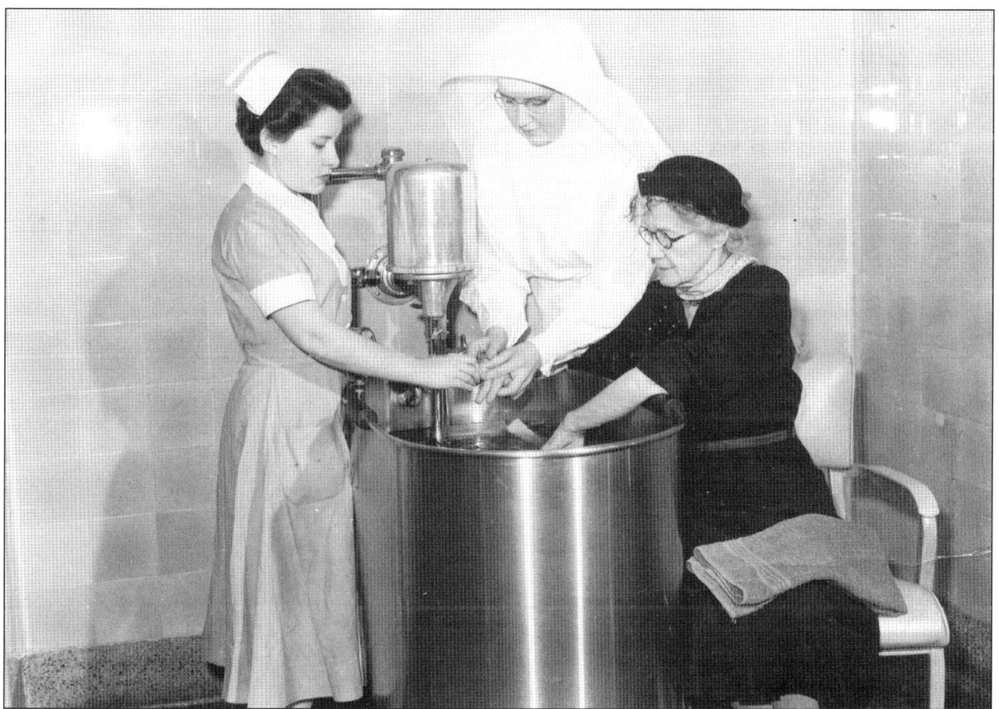

Sr. Pauline Brecanier teaches a student nurse how to provide therapy to a resident. Rehabilitation has been an important component of care in Carmelite homes since the 1950s.

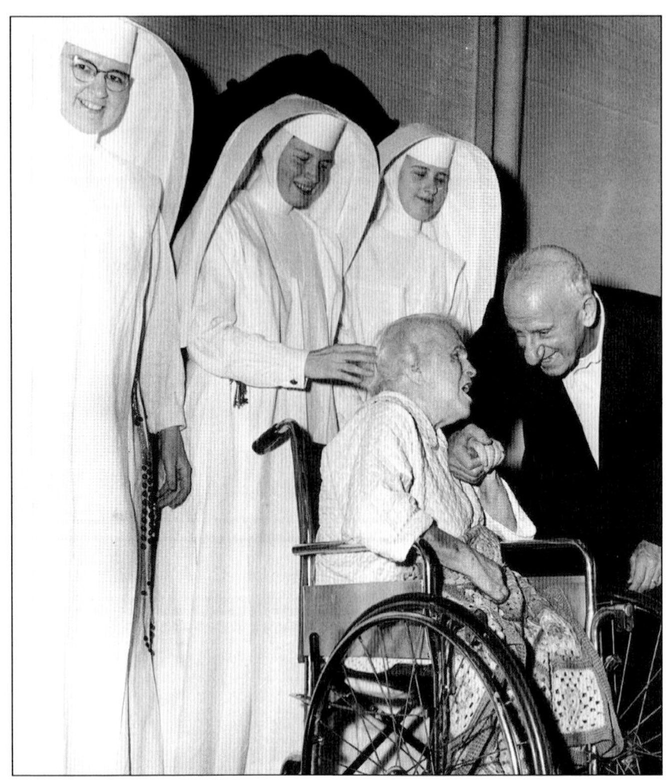

Standing from left to right, Sr. Pauline Brecanier, Sr. Elizabeth Mary, and Sr. Thérèse of the Infant Jesus are seen here with a resident being greeted by Jimmy Durante, a frequent visitor to the sisters' homes in New York City.

On the right is Mother Alodie, one of Mother Angeline's original companions; she was the first administrator of Sacred Heart Manor in Germantown, Pennsylvania, when it was acquired by the Carmelite Sisters in 1937. Here, she is seen with another sister and two residents.

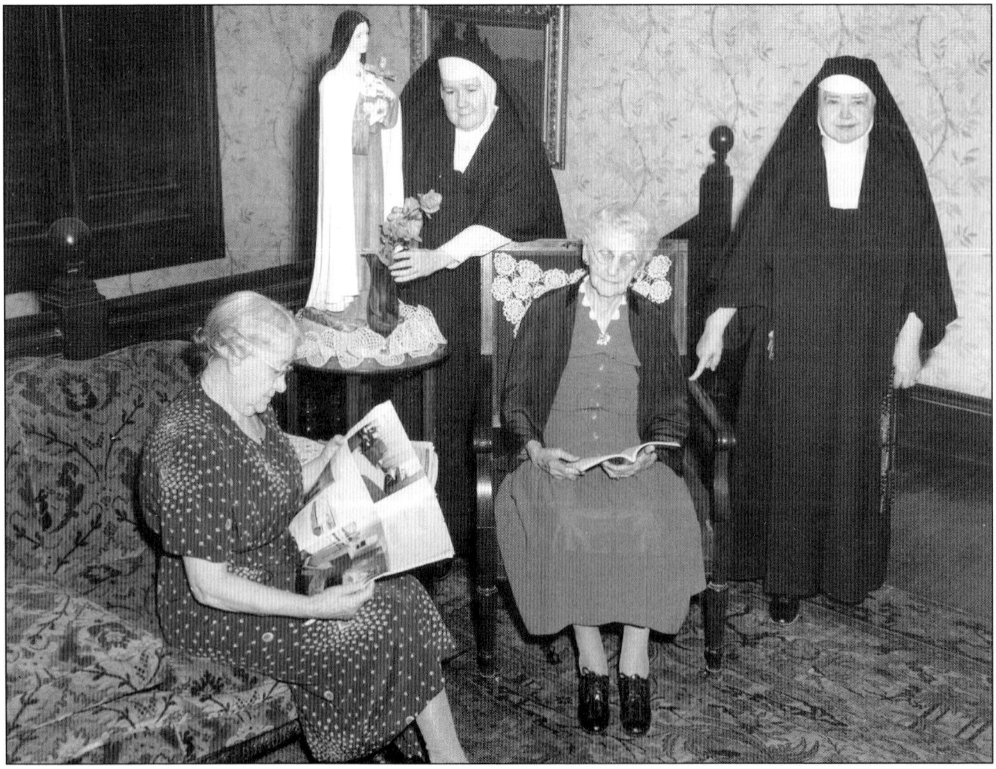

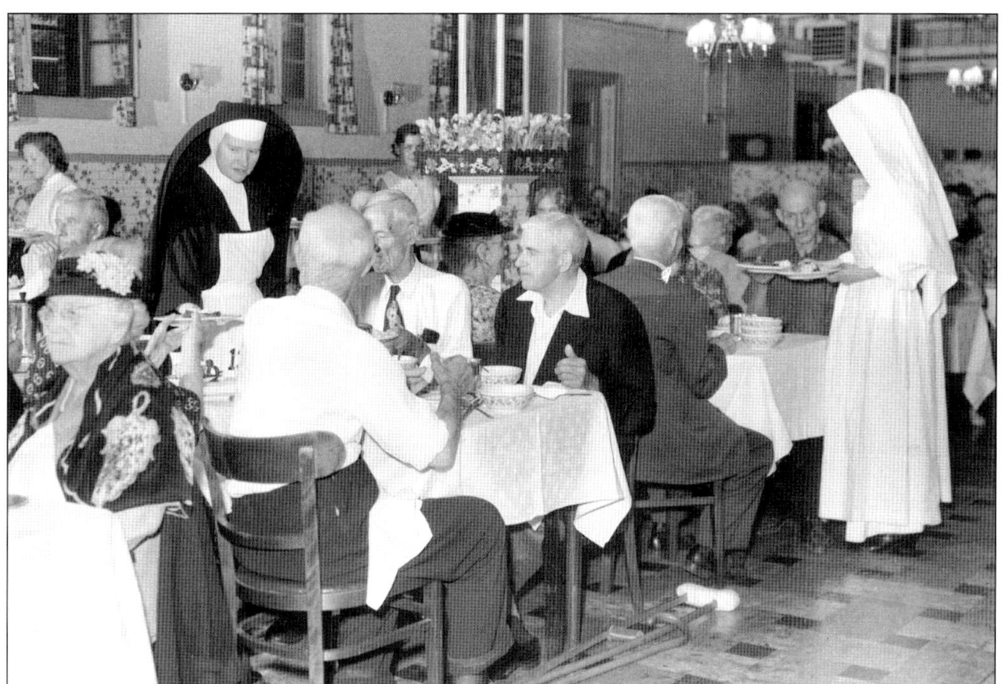

Sr. Daniel of the Blessed Sacrament ministered in social work for many years at St. Patrick's Home. Behind her and to the left, a Carmelette (high school volunteer) can be seen serving the residents.

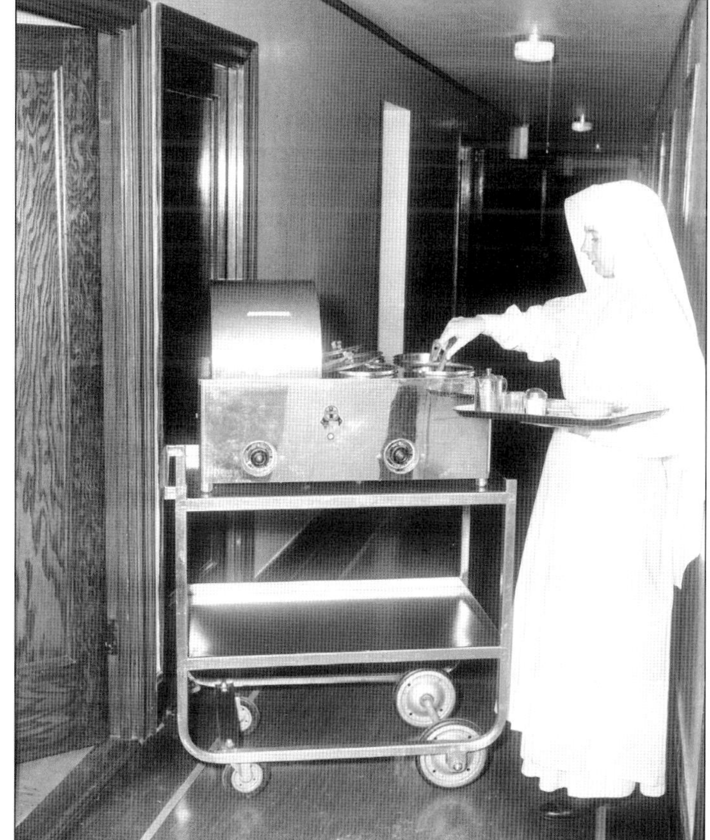

A sister at St. Patrick's Home is preparing a tray for a bedridden resident. Hall carts were used to keep the food hot for those residents who could not get to the dining room.

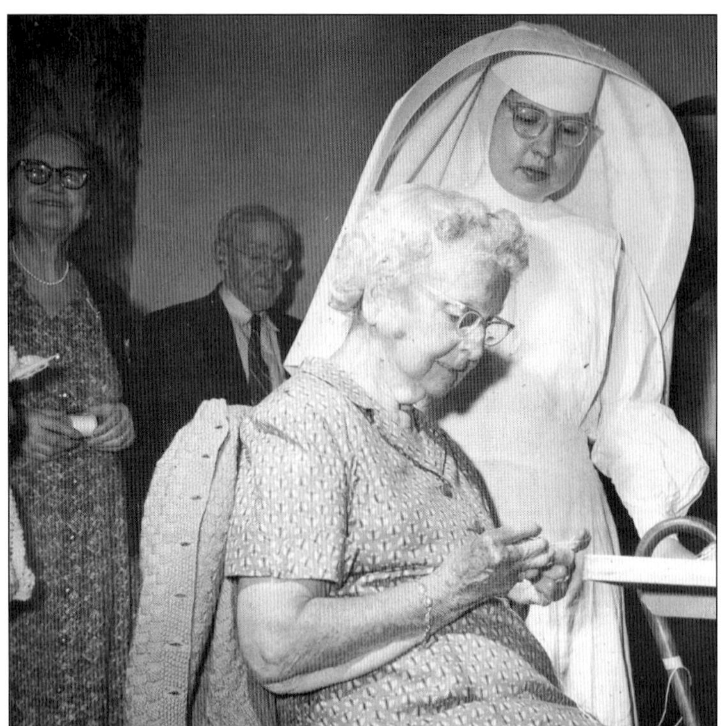

Sr. Elena Castaneda provides an occupational therapy treatment to a resident.

Sr. Patricia of the Queen of Carmel and a postulant read a resident's Christmas cards to her. The holidays can be a lonely time for residents, and they appreciate extra care and attention at that time.

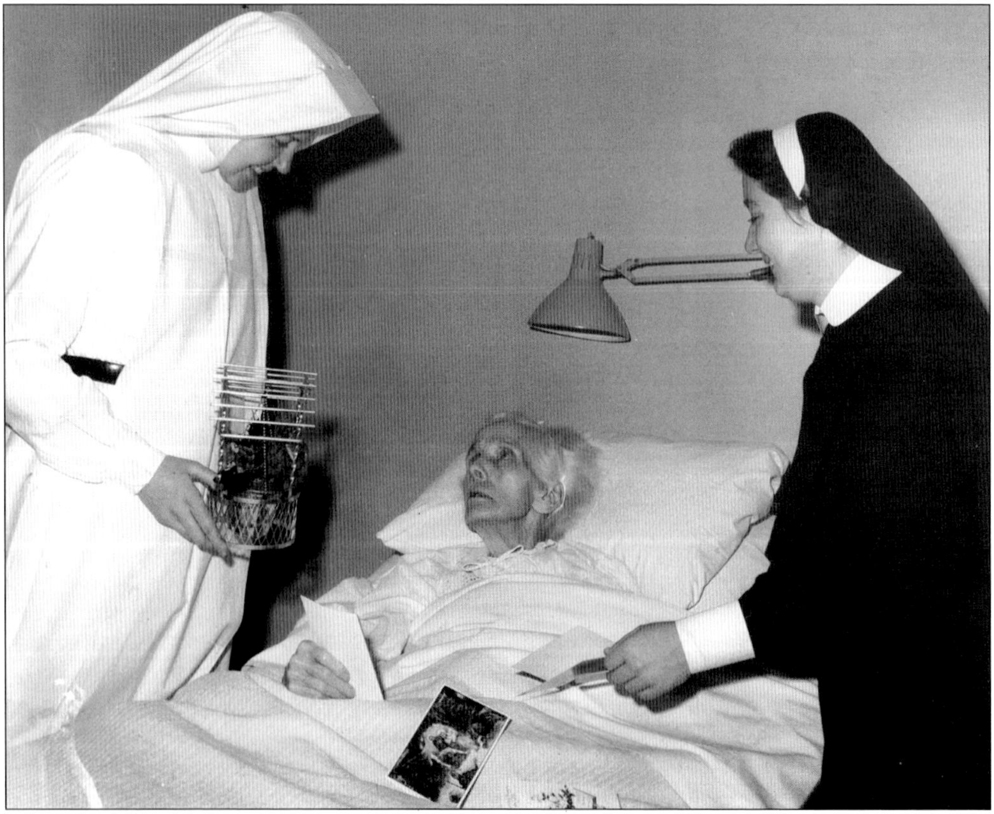

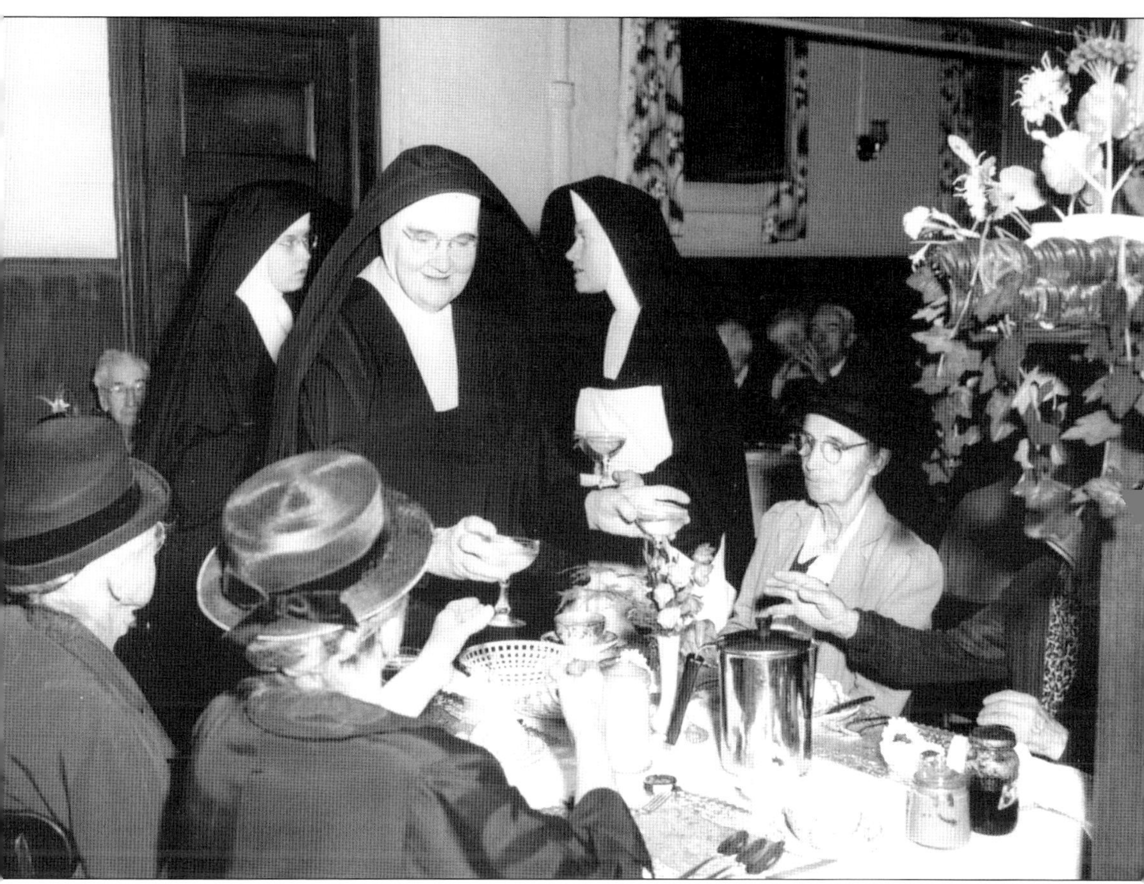

In spite of her busy schedule as superior general, whenever Mother Angeline visited one of the facilities, she would always spend time with the residents. In this photograph, she is serving wine to residents.

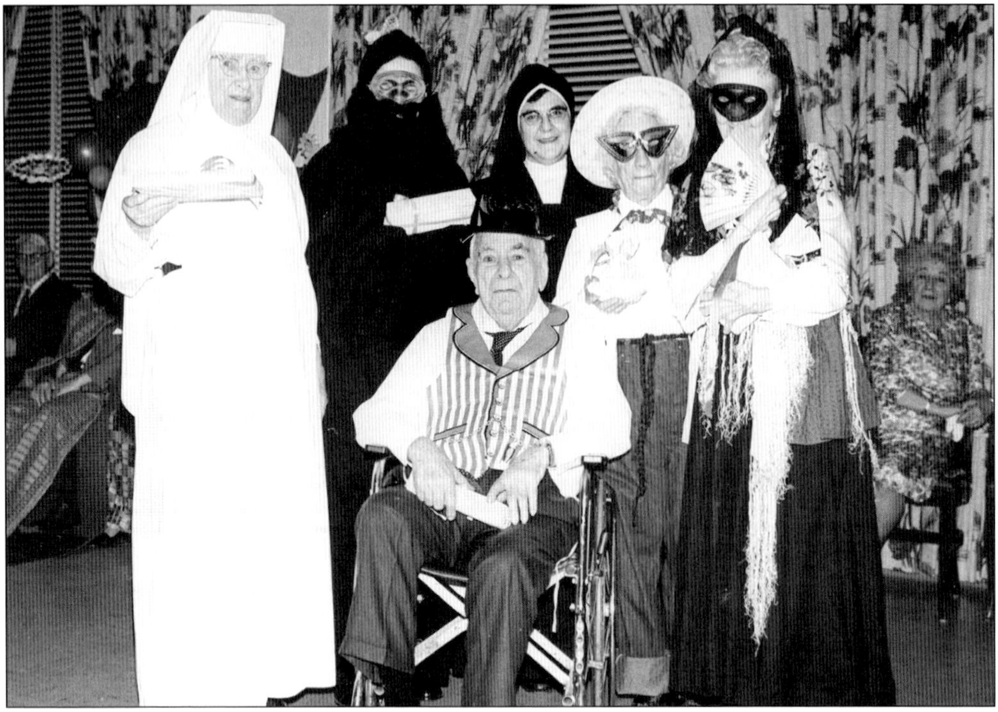

Sr. Mary Ellen Bernadette and another sister helped these residents at Mary Manning Walsh get ready to party for Mardi Gras.

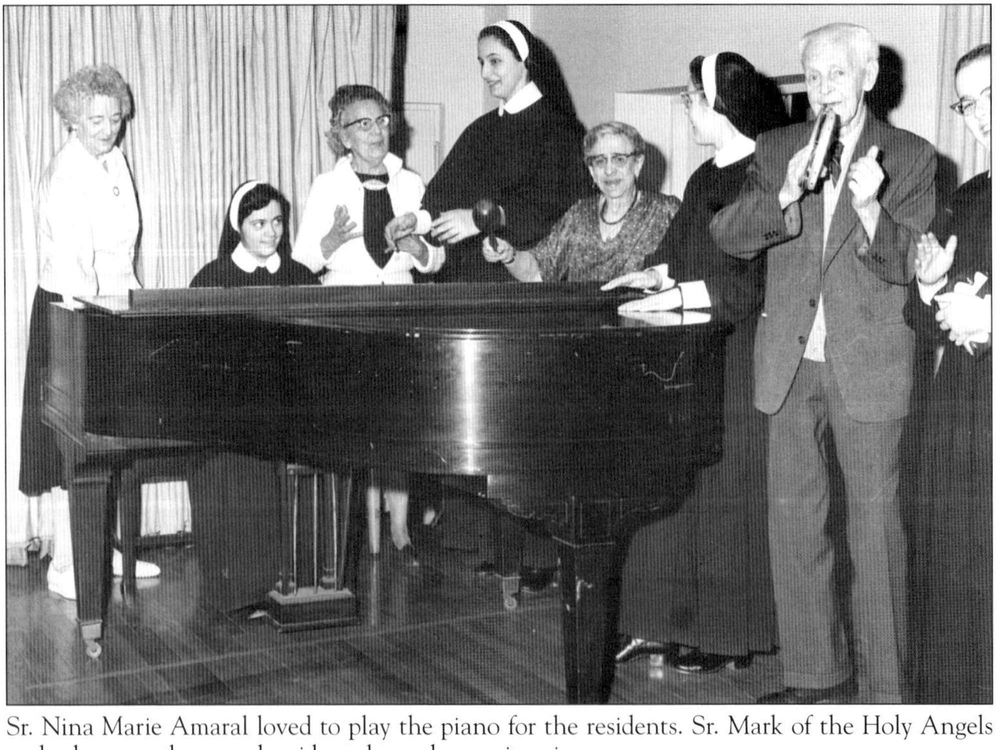

Sr. Nina Marie Amaral loved to play the piano for the residents. Sr. Mark of the Holy Angels and other postulants and residents keep the music going.

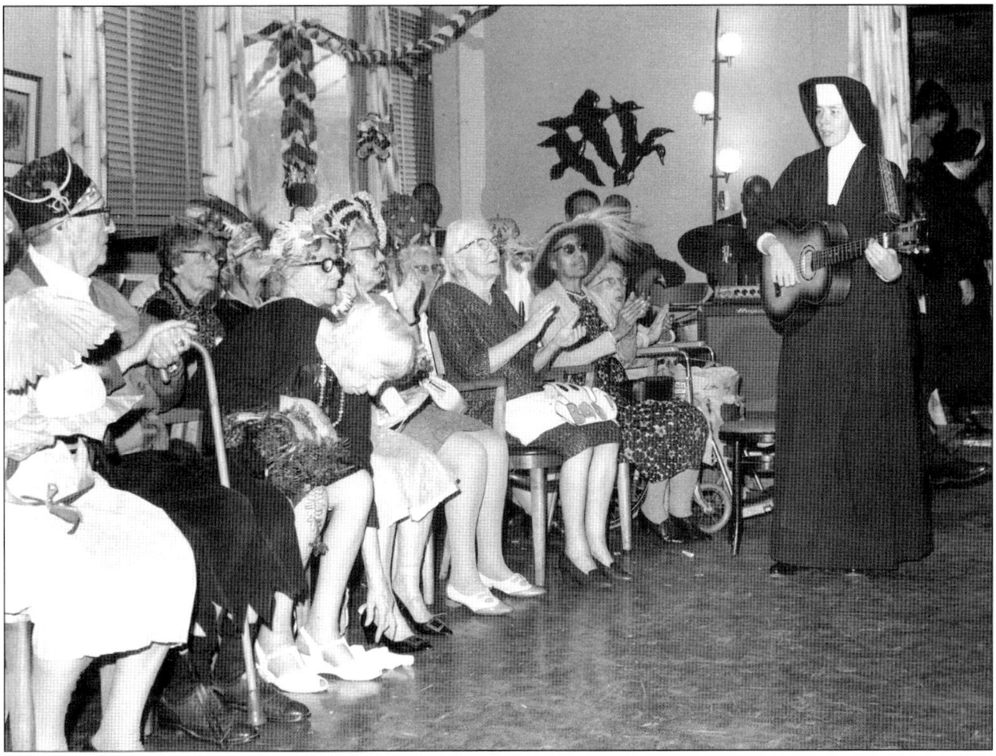

Sr. Imelda De Lourdes loved to entertain the residents with her guitar for sing-along sessions.

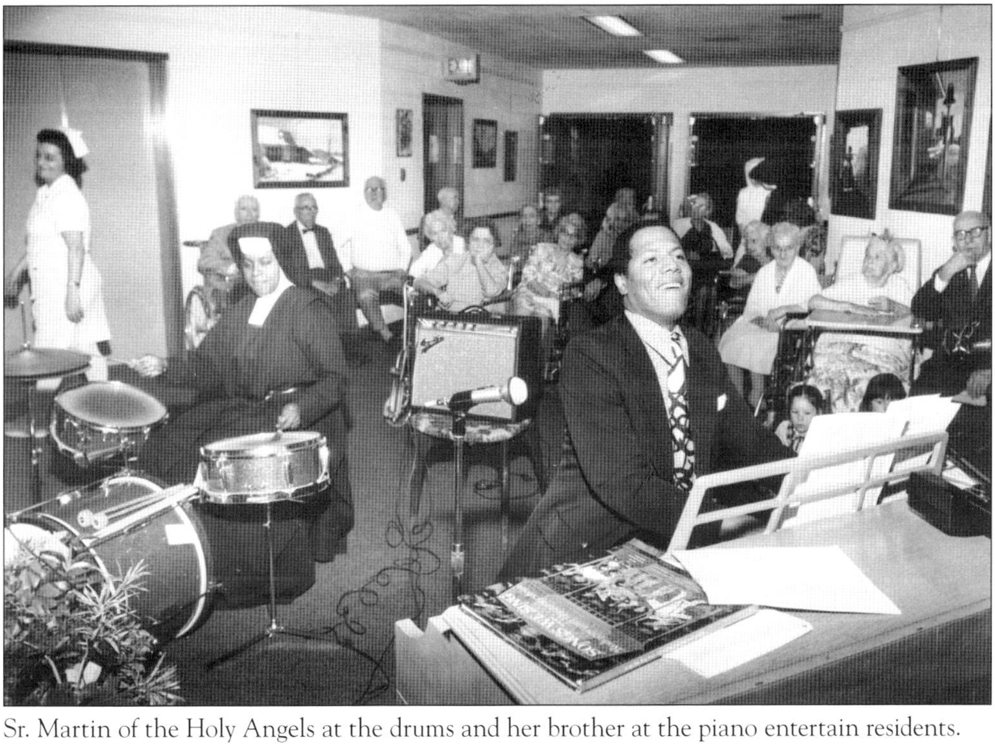

Sr. Martin of the Holy Angels at the drums and her brother at the piano entertain residents.

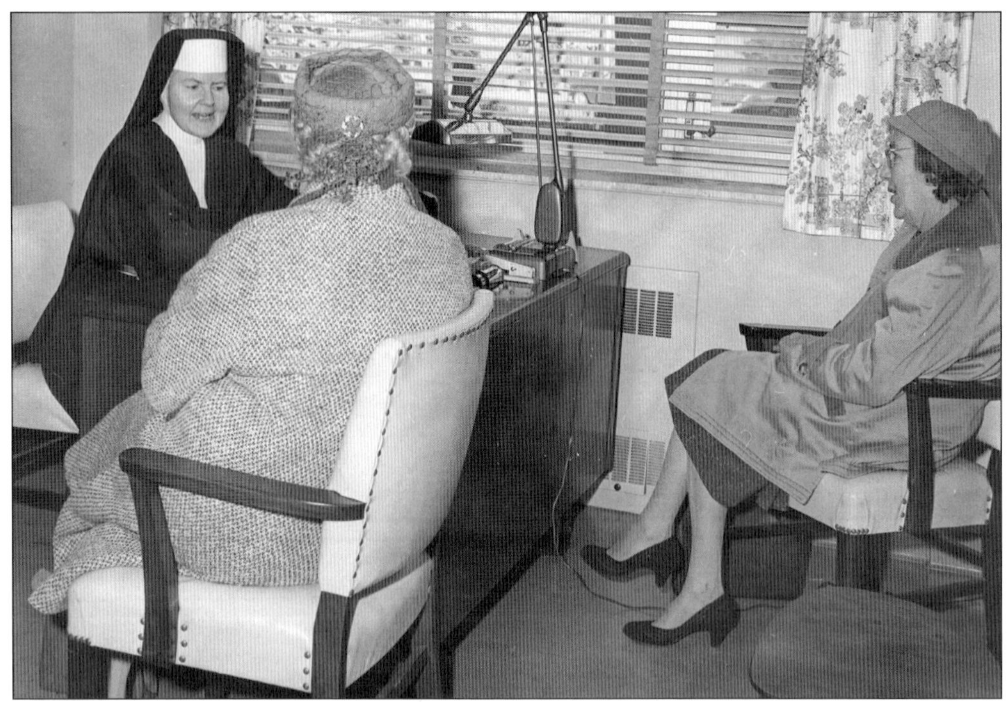

Sr. M. John Joseph served for many years as a licensed social worker at Mary Manning Walsh Home in New York City and St. Joseph's Manor in Trumbull, Connecticut. Here, she is seen interviewing a resident.

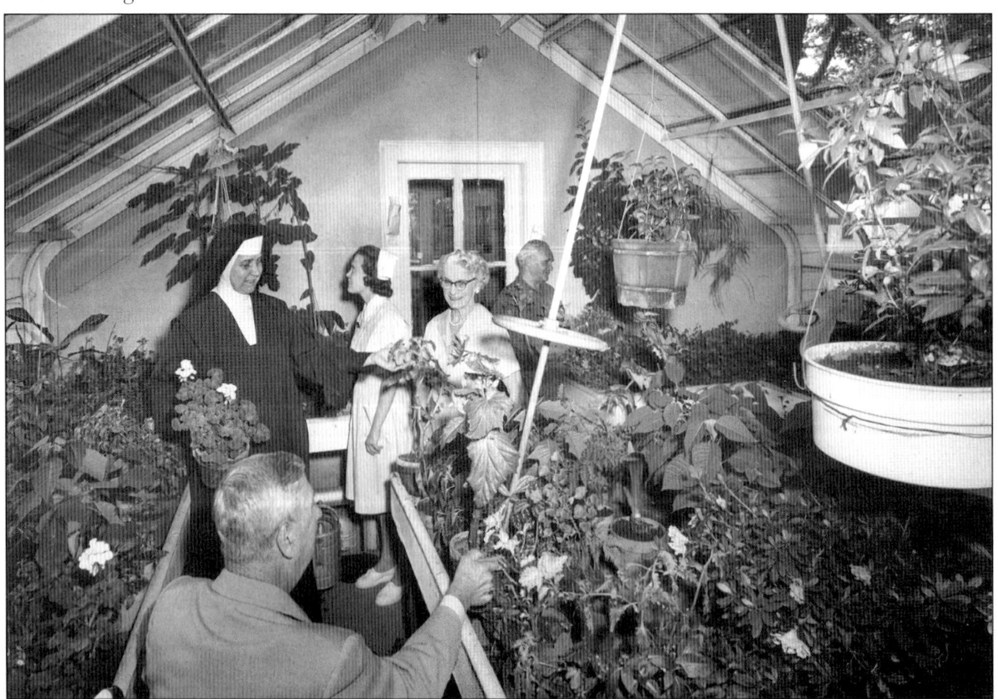

Sr. M. Carmelita of the Infant Jesus is seen taking a break from her work as financial manager in the business office to show residents the greenhouse at St. Joseph's Manor in Trumbull, Connecticut.

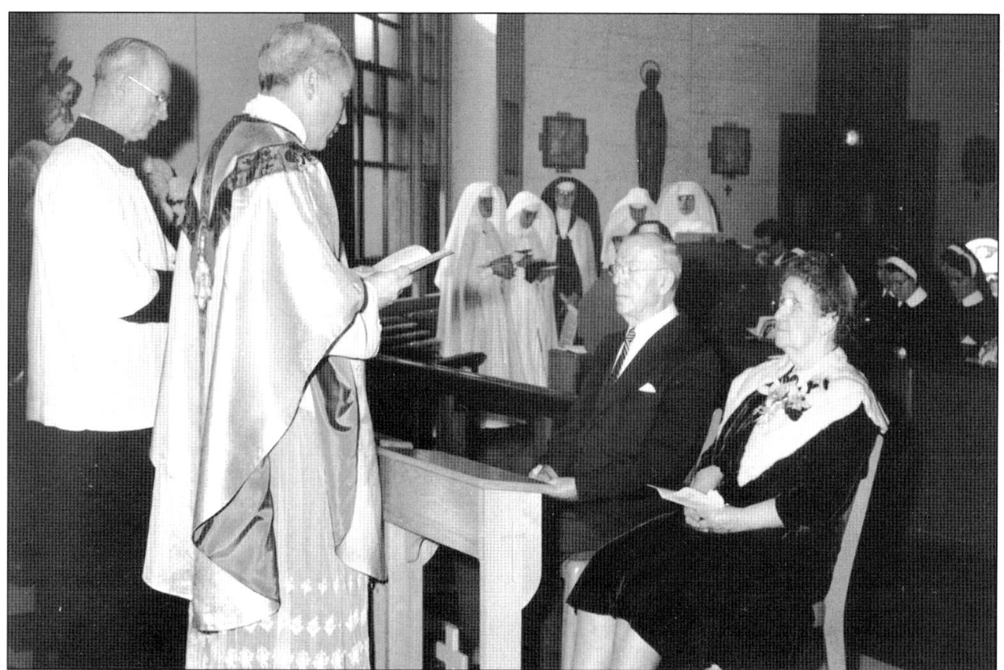

Residents are renewing their vows for their 50th anniversary. From the early days, Mother Angeline insisted that married couples be allowed to stay together when they became residents of a Carmelite nursing home. It is standard today, but was revolutionary in those days.

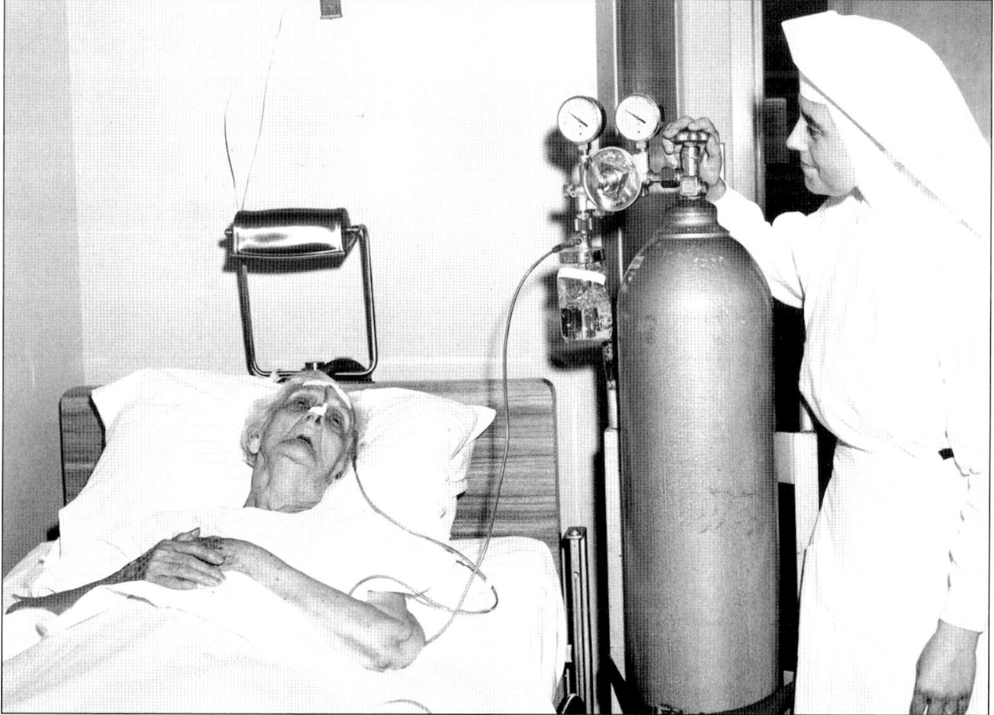

Always attentive to the needs of residents and their families, Sr. Patrick of the Assumption checks the levels in the oxygen tank of a resident confined to bed.

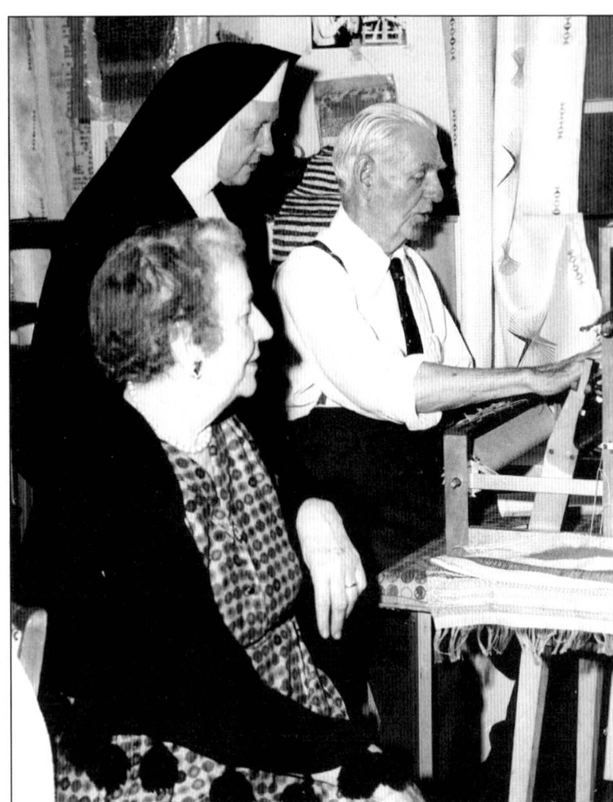

Sr. Alodie Therese watches as residents of Josephine Baird Nursing home show her how to work a loom.

Sr. Joseph Michael is pictured with a Carmelette and residents on the rooftop shuffleboard court at Josephine Baird Nursing Home.

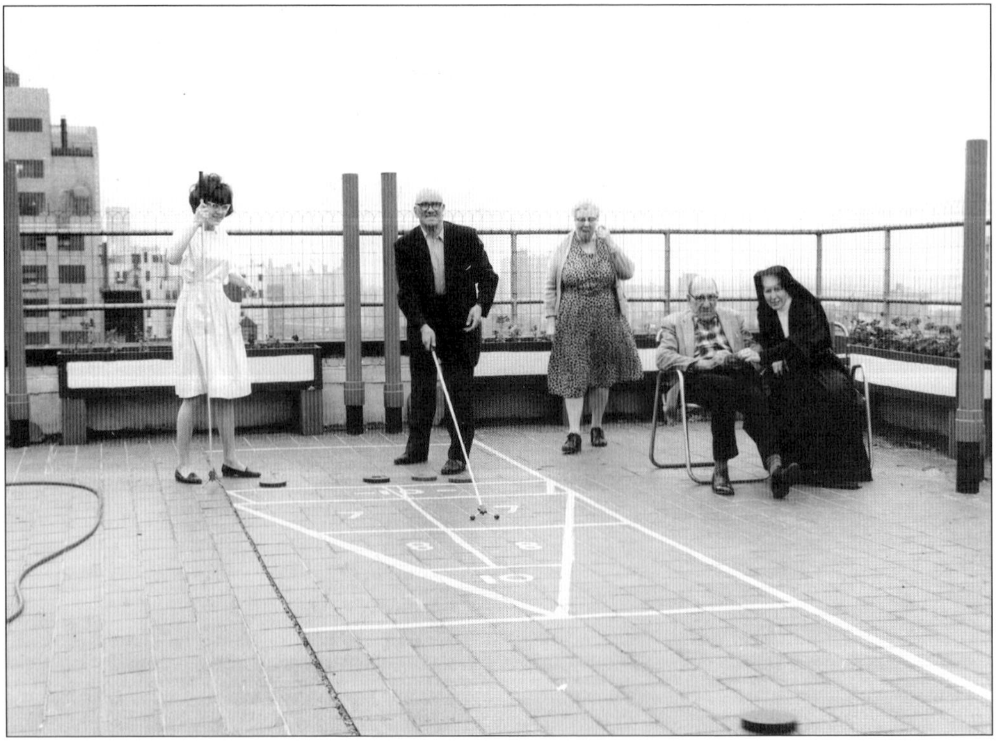

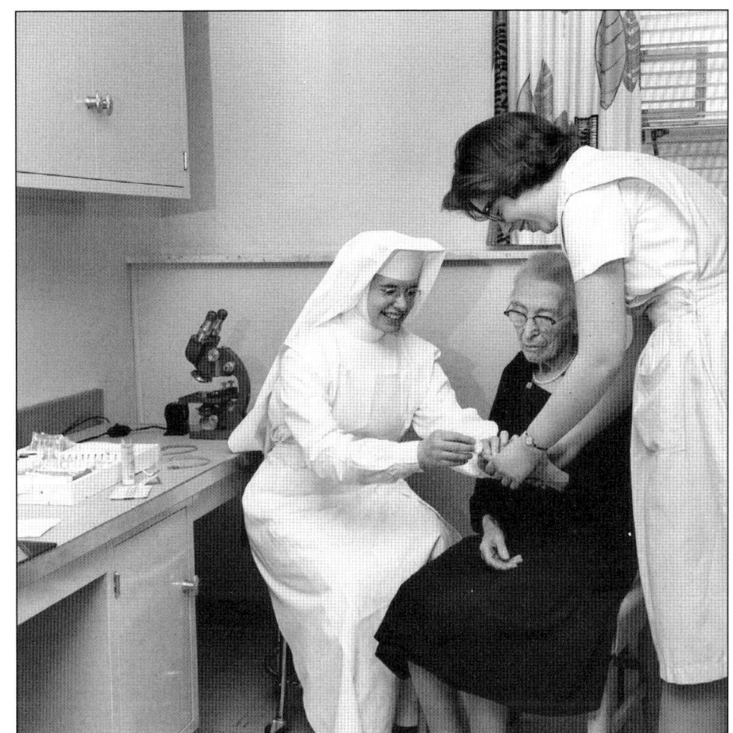

Sr. Christopher of the Queen of Carmel takes a blood sample from a resident at St. Joseph's Manor in Trumbull, Connecticut, with the assistance of a Carmelette.

Sr. Brian of All Saints and two nurses help residents blow out the candles on their birthday cake.

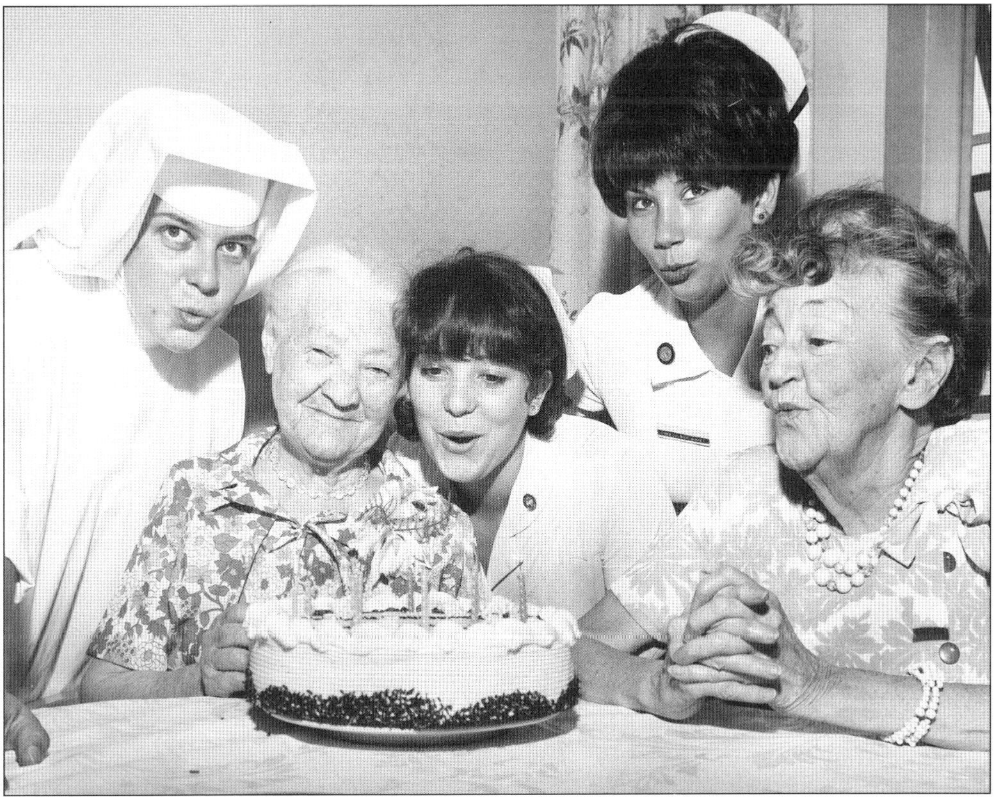

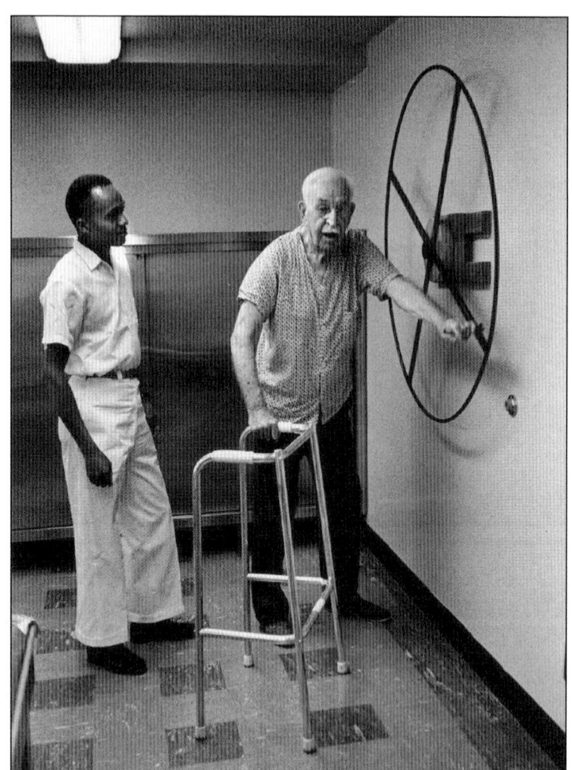

Under the watchful eye of a rehabilitation assistant, a resident uses the therapy wheel at Mary Manning Walsh Home in New York City to recover strength after a stroke.

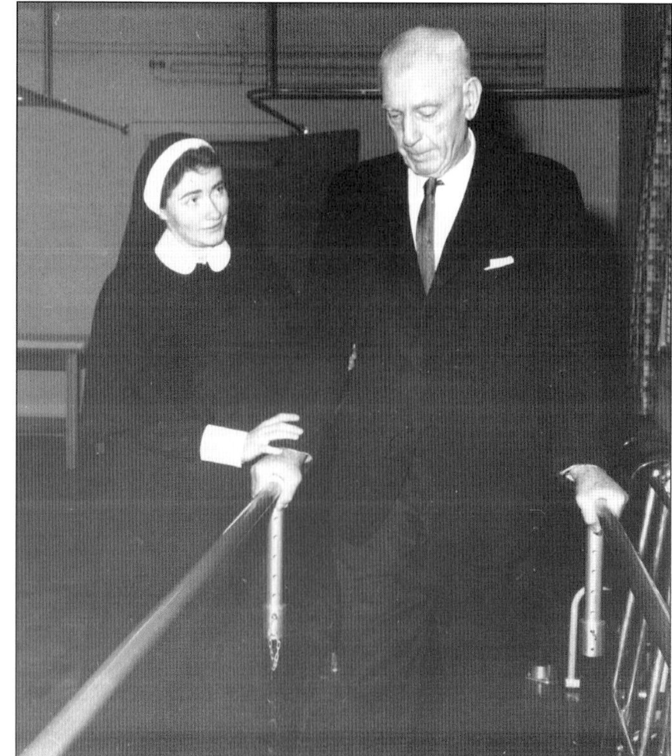

A postulant helps a resident practice walking again after surgery. Postulants serve alongside the professed sisters and learn how to help the residents from them.

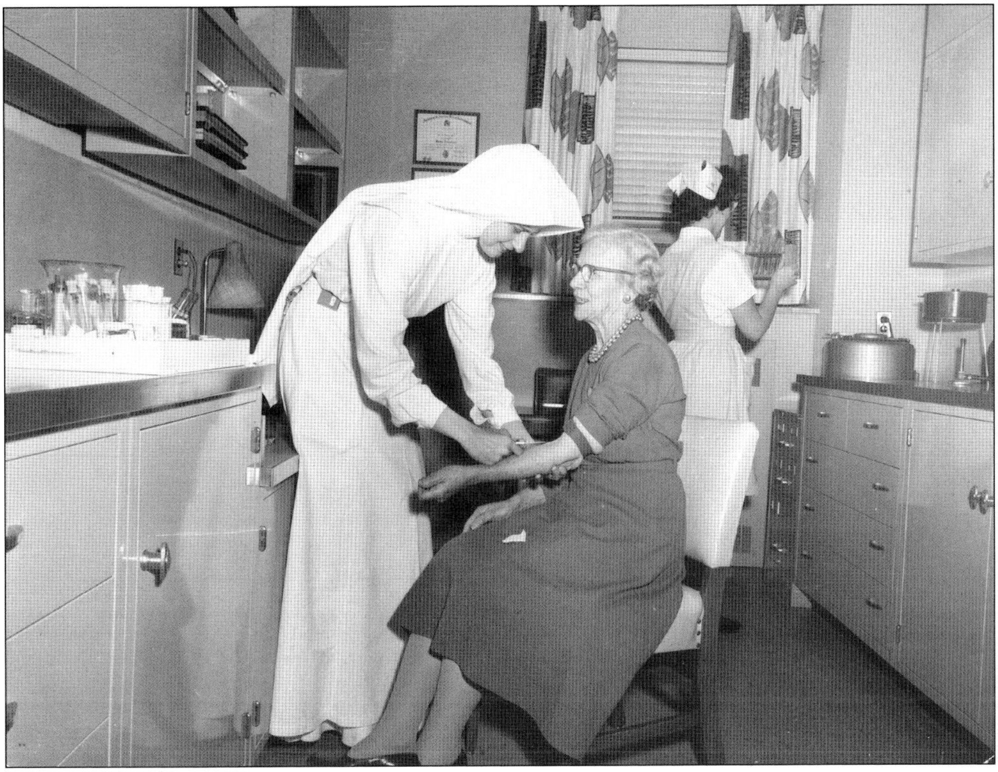

Sr. David Ann De Lourdes takes a blood sample from a resident at St. Joseph's Manor in Trumbull, Connecticut.

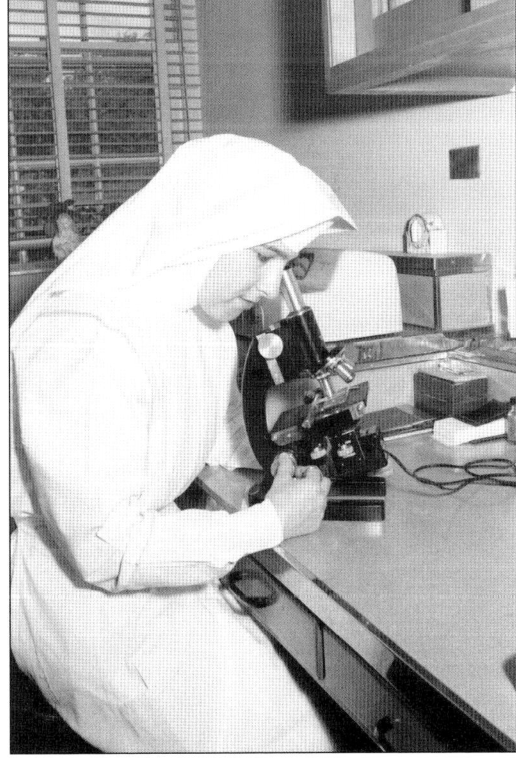

Sr. Therese Mary, seen here at the microscope, trained as a laboratory and X-ray technician. She was so good at reading X-rays that doctors often asked for her opinion.

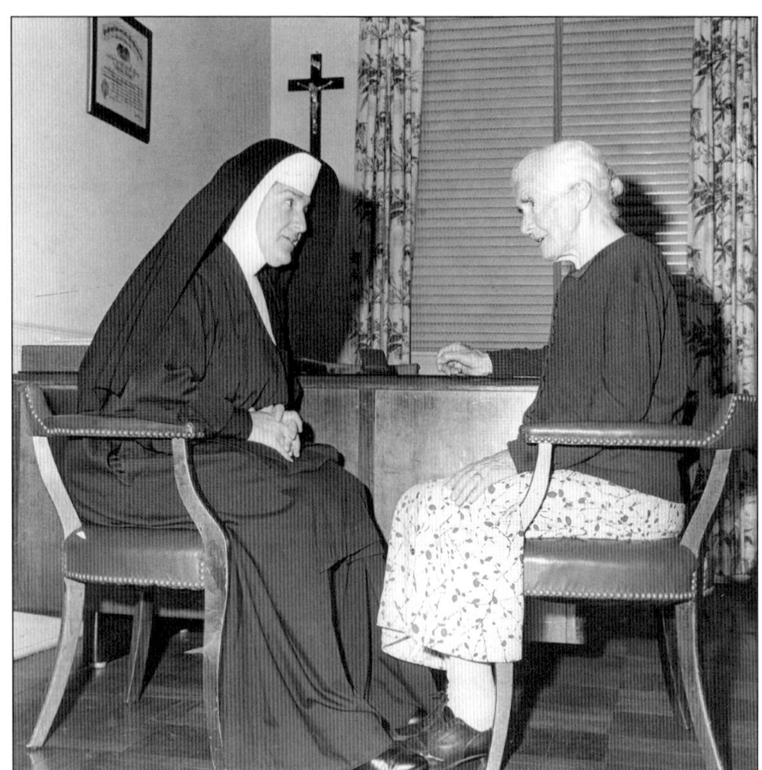

Sr. Maria Jude, social worker, is deep in discussion with a resident.

Sr. Mary Elizabeth Marciano was a licensed social worker. Here, she is seen taking information to admit a resident.

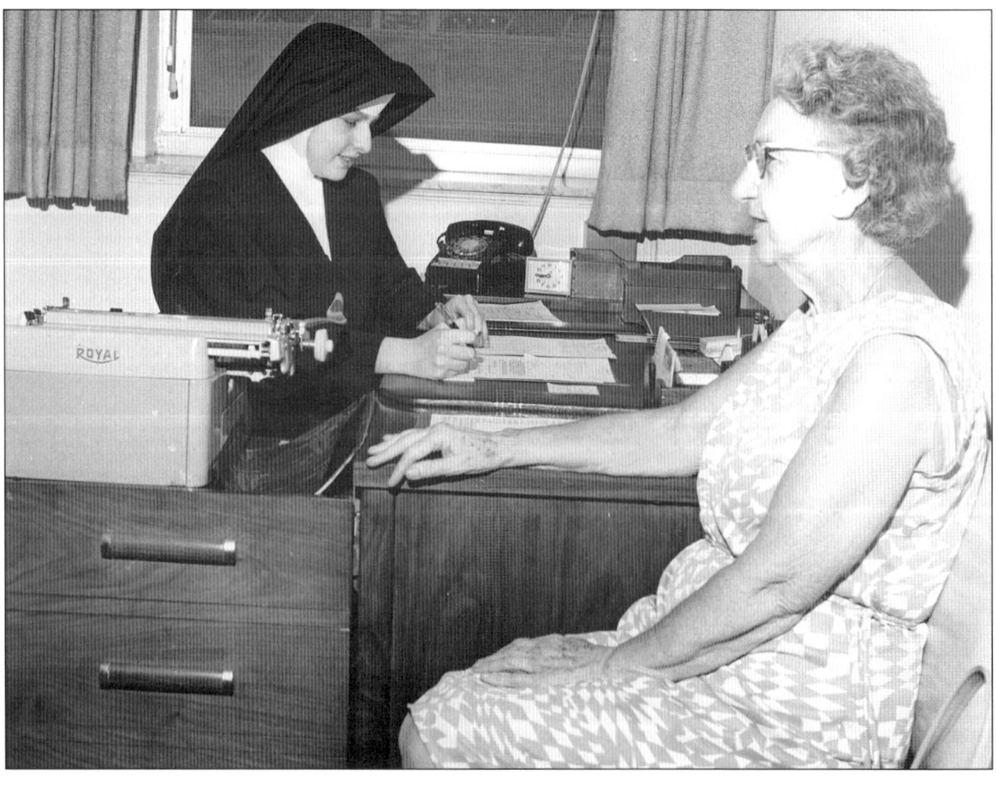

From left to right, Sr. Imelda Regina, Sr. Therese Patricia, and Sr. Juliette Marie prepare a treat for the residents in the kitchen of Saint Joseph's Manor.

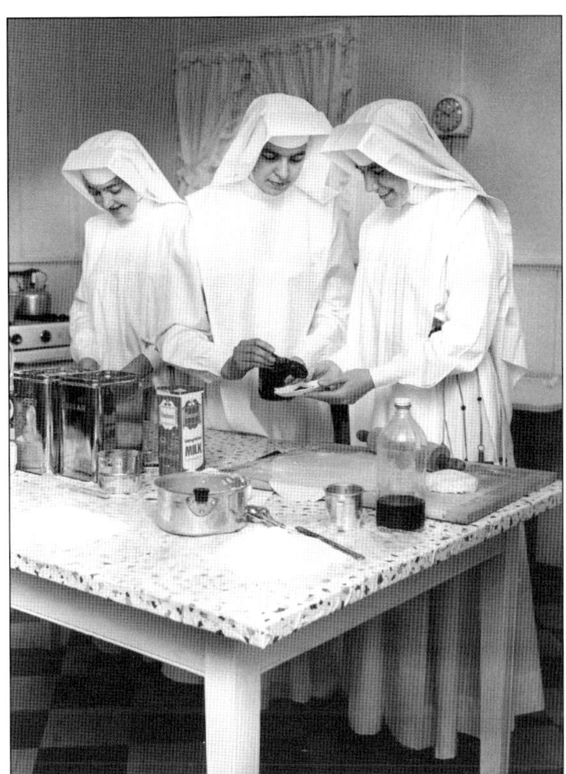

Mother Marie de Lourdes and a postulant serve beverages to the residents in the dining room.

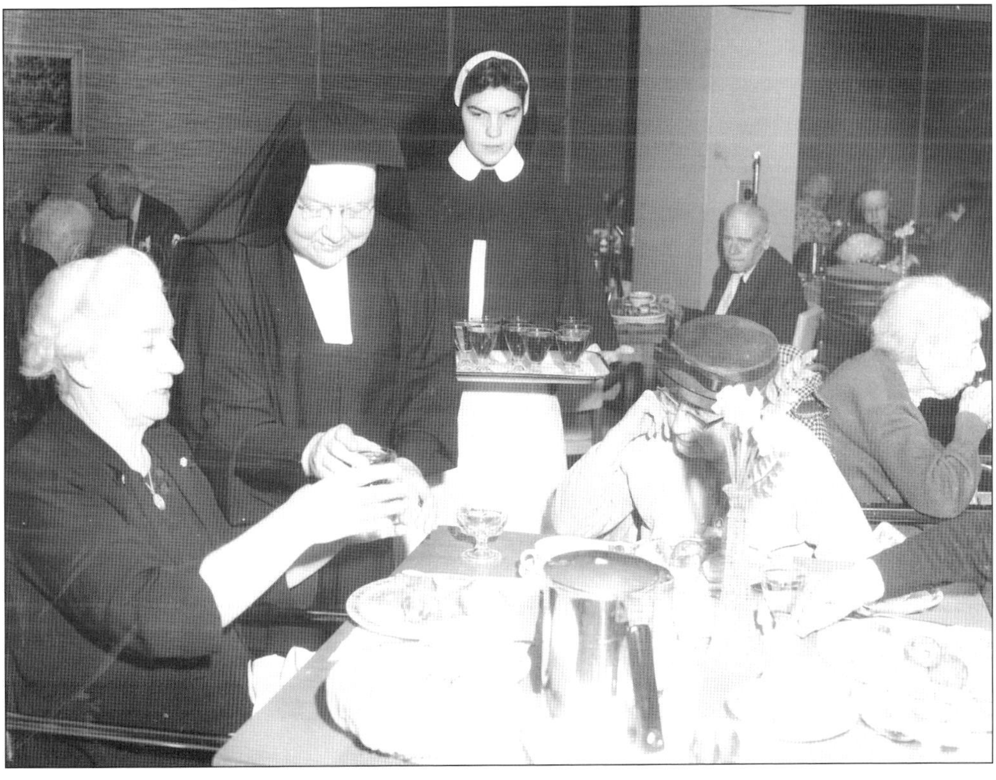

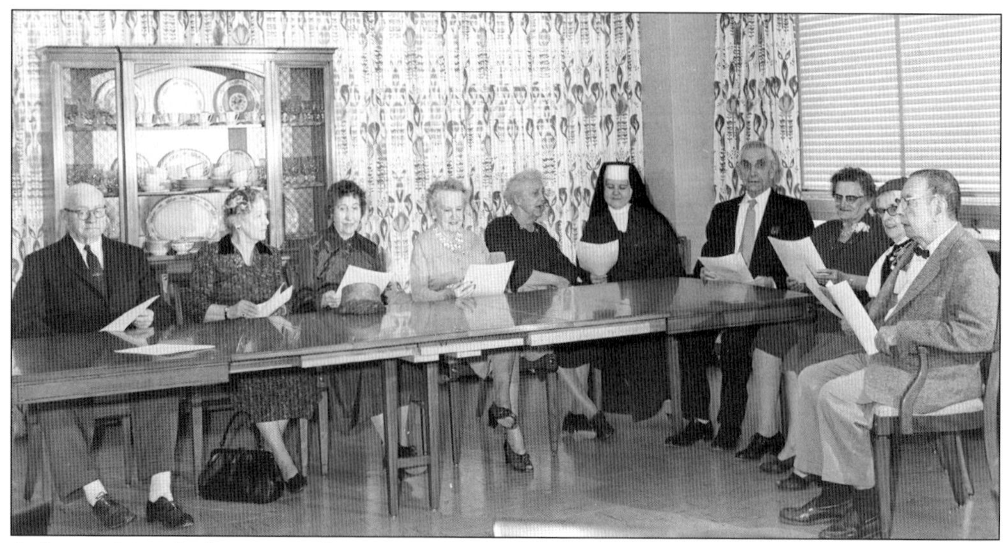

Sr. Jacinta Mary facilitates a resident council meeting at St. Joseph's Manor in Trumbull, Connecticut. Carmelite homes established resident councils in the 1950s to give residents a voice in their care.

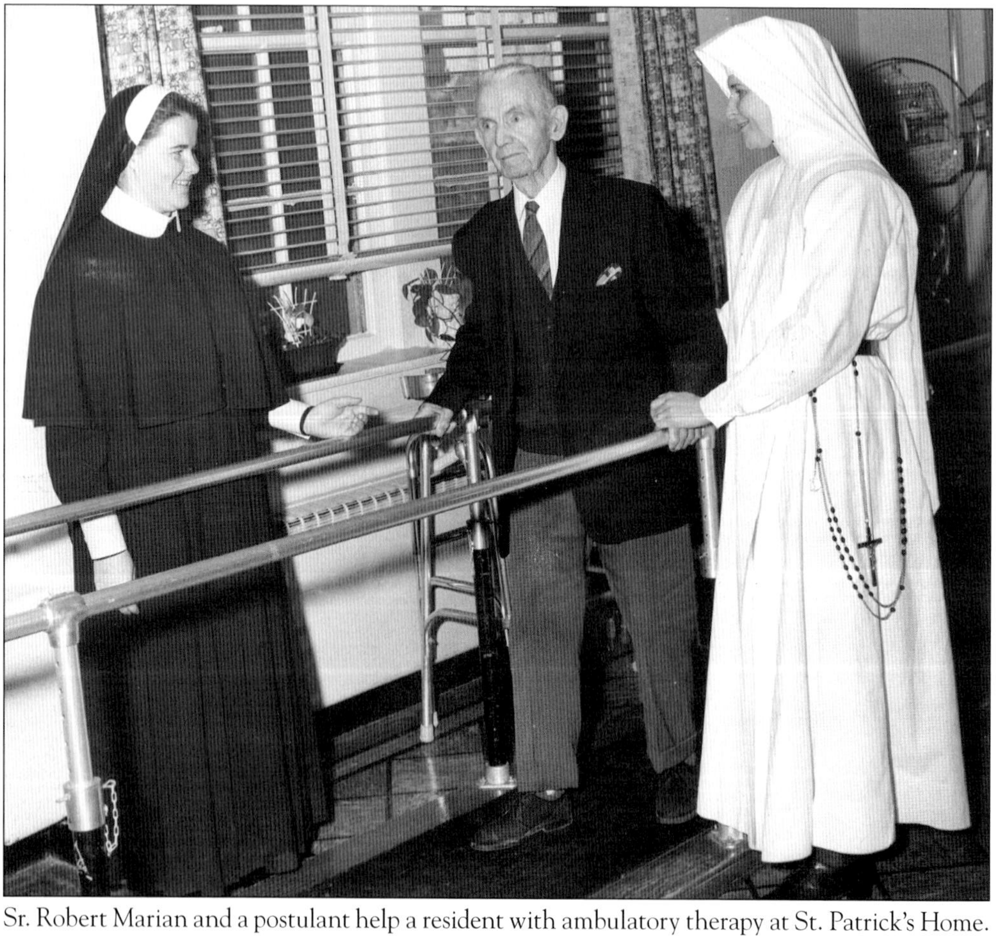

Sr. Robert Marian and a postulant help a resident with ambulatory therapy at St. Patrick's Home.

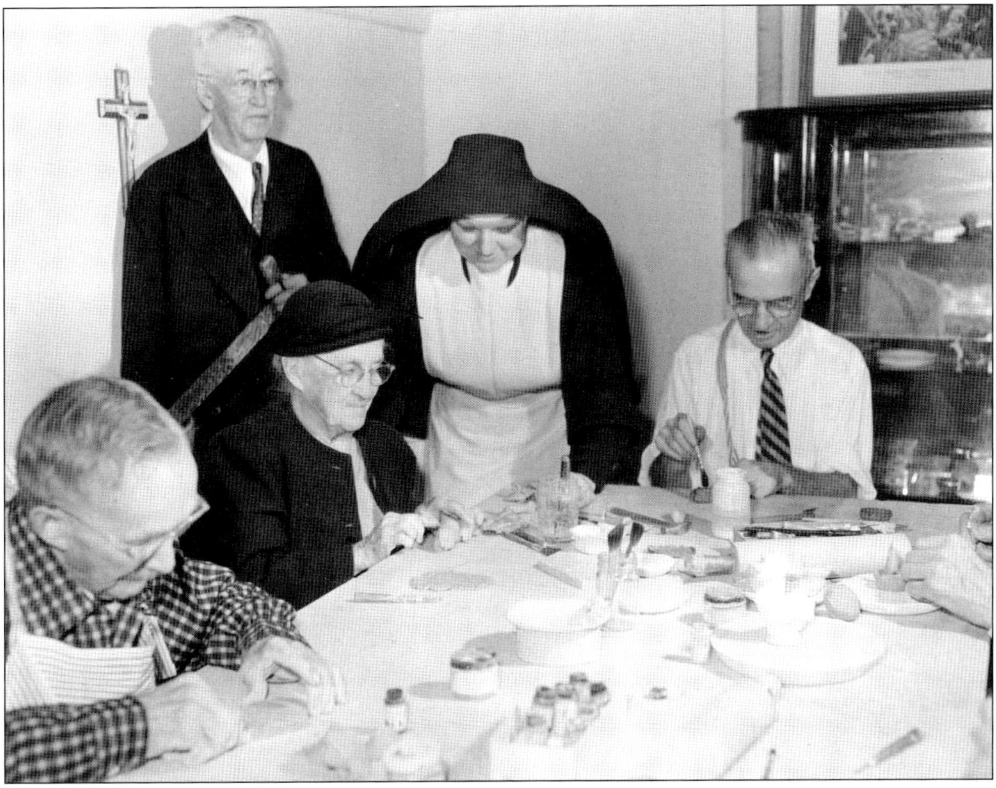

A sister works with residents on their projects in occupational therapy.

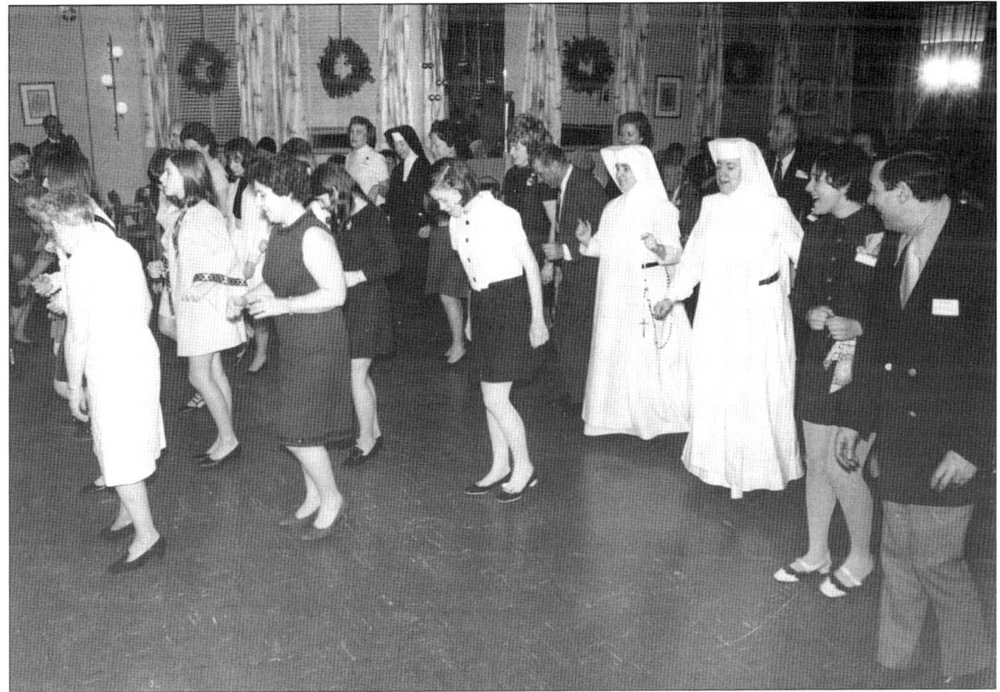

Sisters loved to join in the fun of line dancing, to the amusement of the residents.

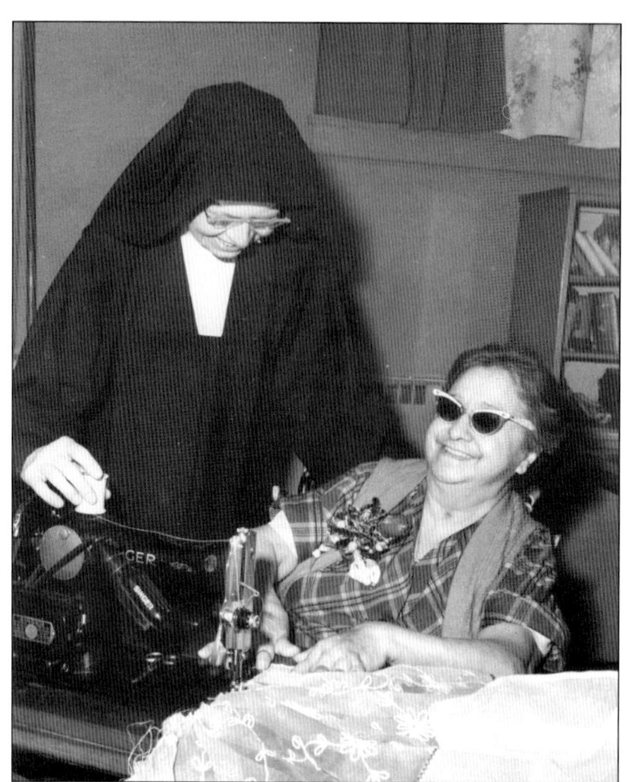

Sr. Charles of St. Joseph encourages a resident in her sewing project. She was an accomplished calligrapher who loved working with the residents.

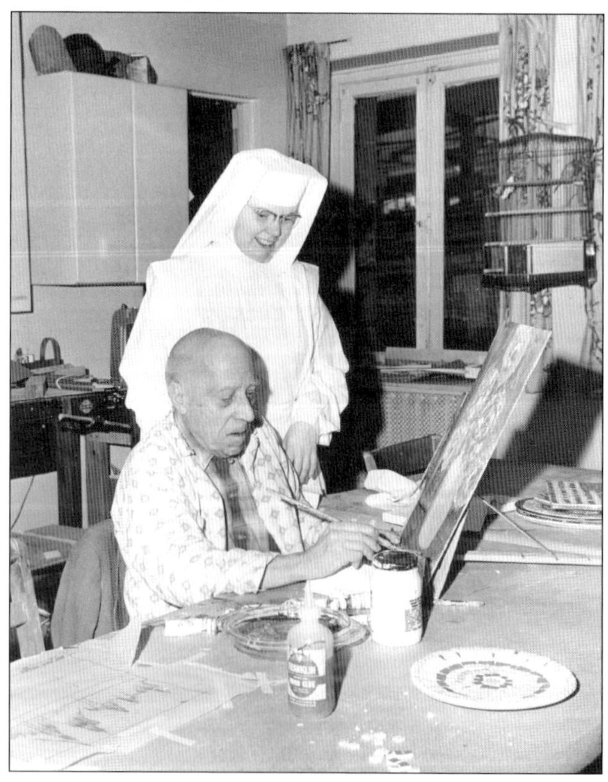

Sr. Celine Marian helps a resident with his painting.

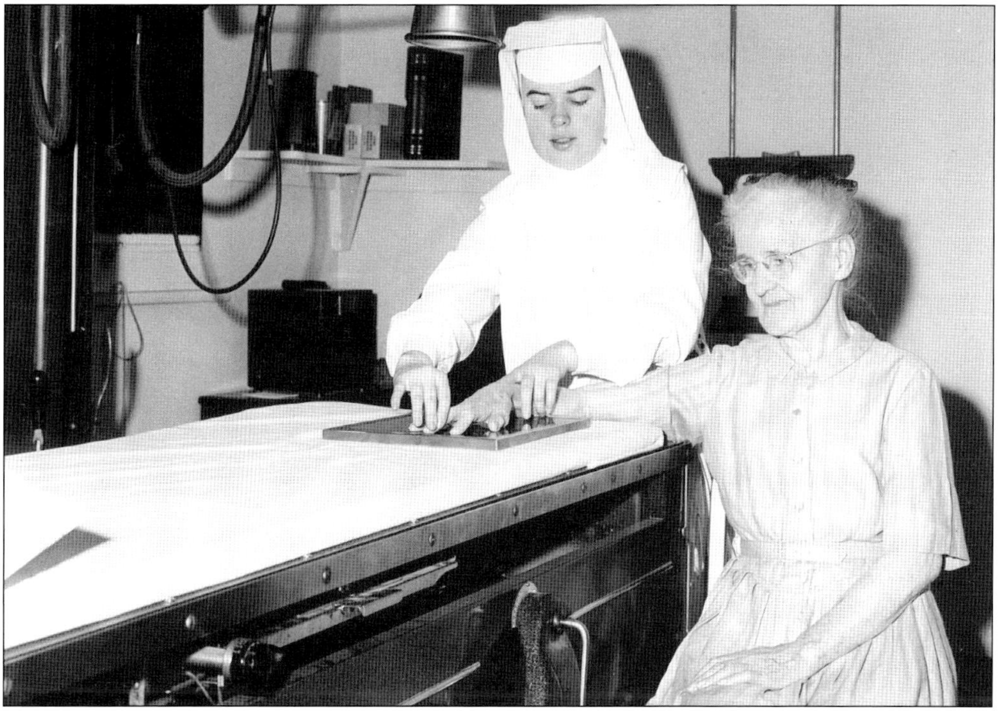

Sr. Margaret Patrick Marie prepares to take an X-ray of the hand of a resident at Saint Patrick's Home.

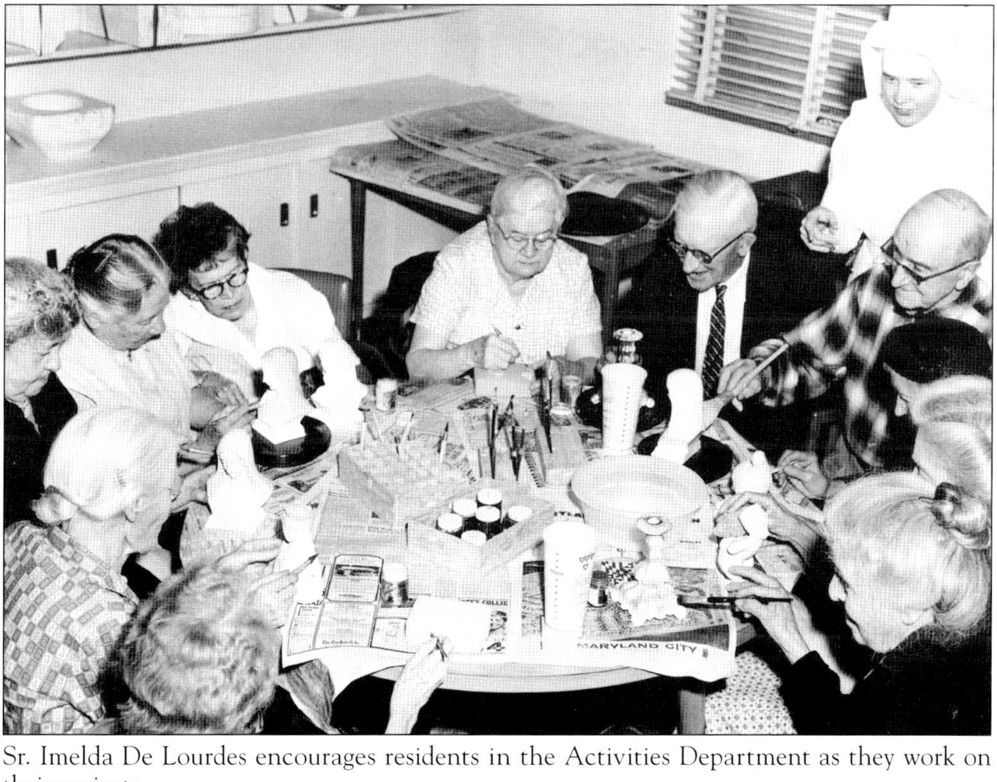

Sr. Imelda De Lourdes encourages residents in the Activities Department as they work on their projects.

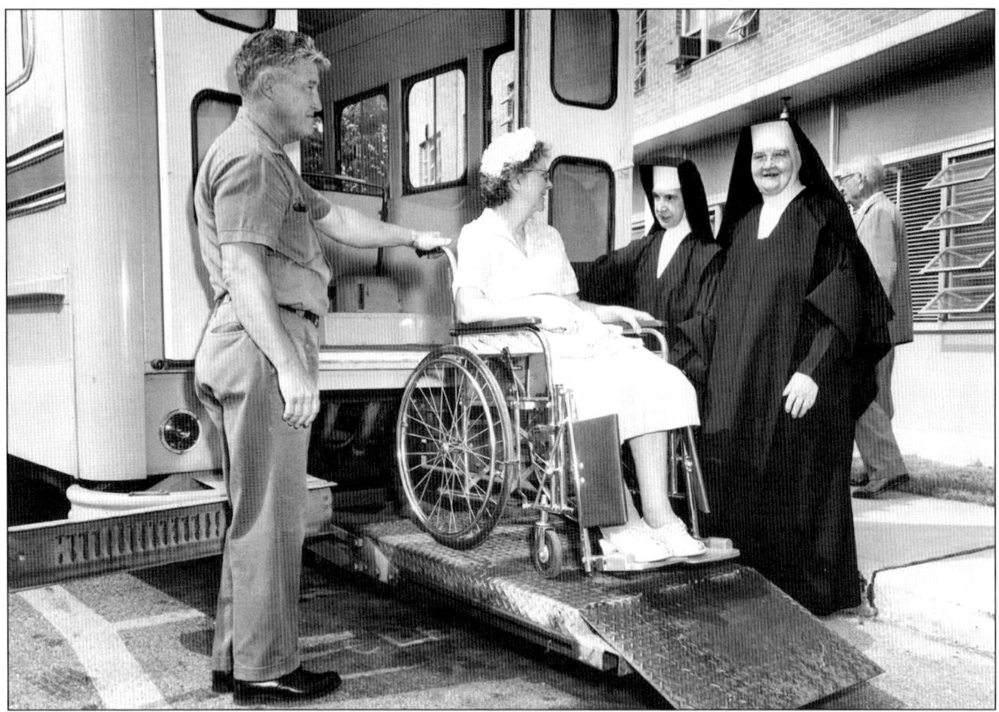

Mother Angeline is in the foreground and Mother Bernadette is behind her as the St. Joseph's Manor van driver shows them how the chair lift functions.

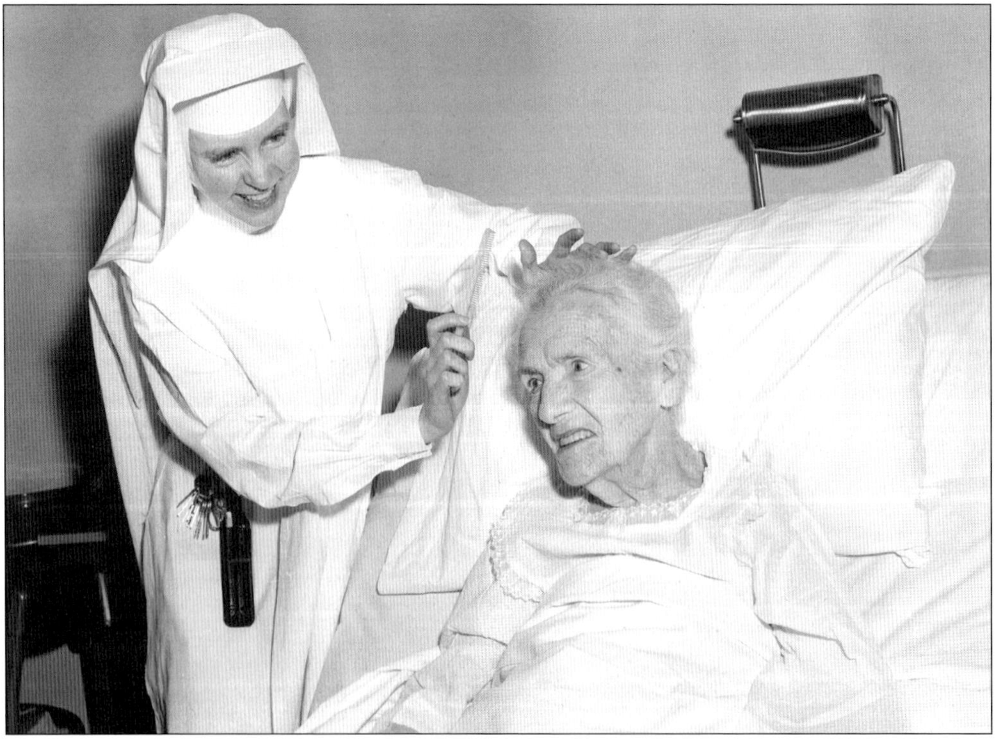

Sr. Agnes Patricia lovingly combs the hair of a bedridden resident.

Sr. Therese Patricia helps a resident remove baked bread from the oven.

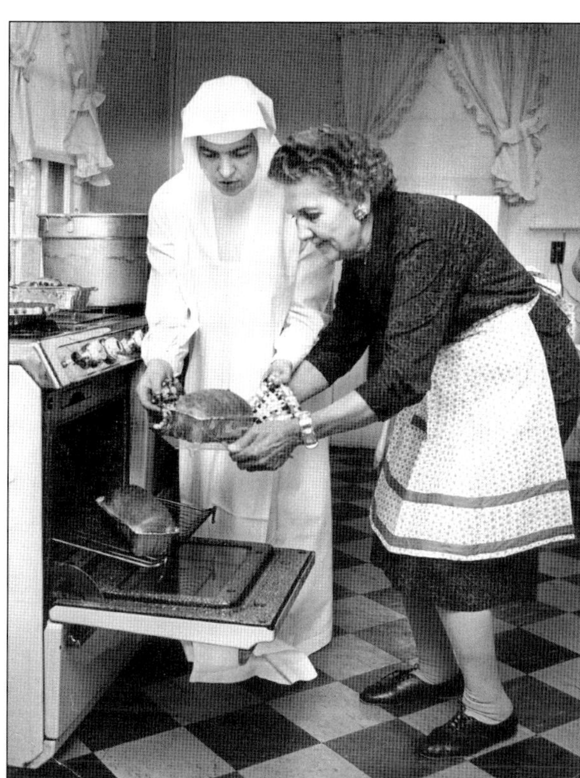

Sr. Serafino, at far left, leads the spirited resident chorus. She shared her extensive musical gifts over the years with residents and sisters alike.

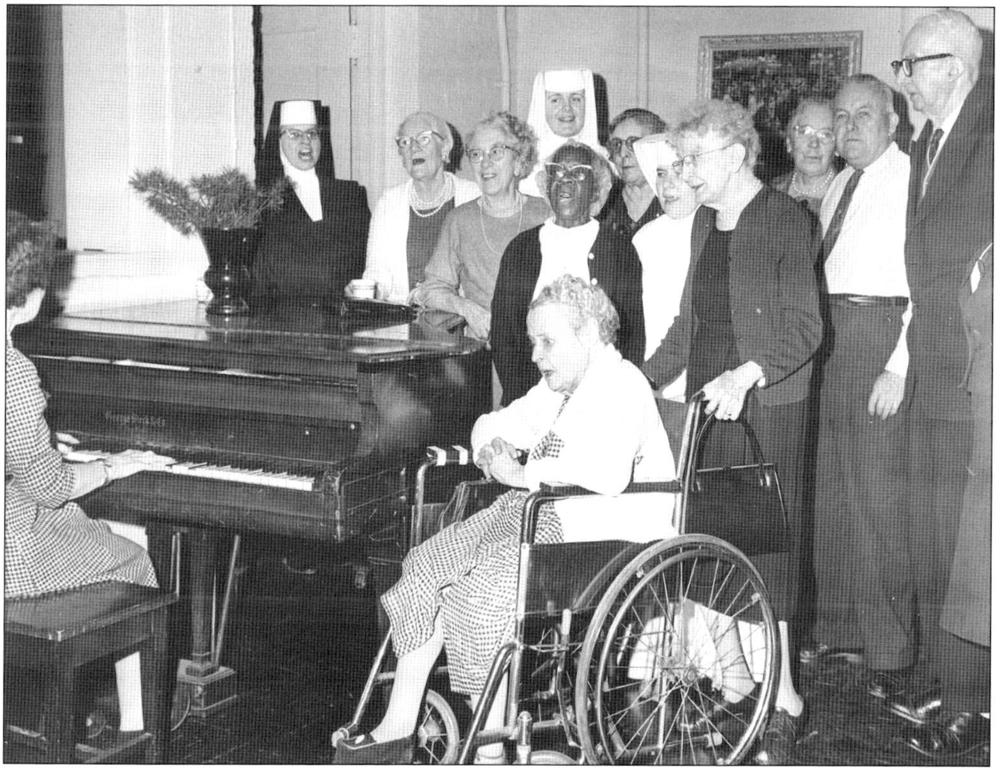

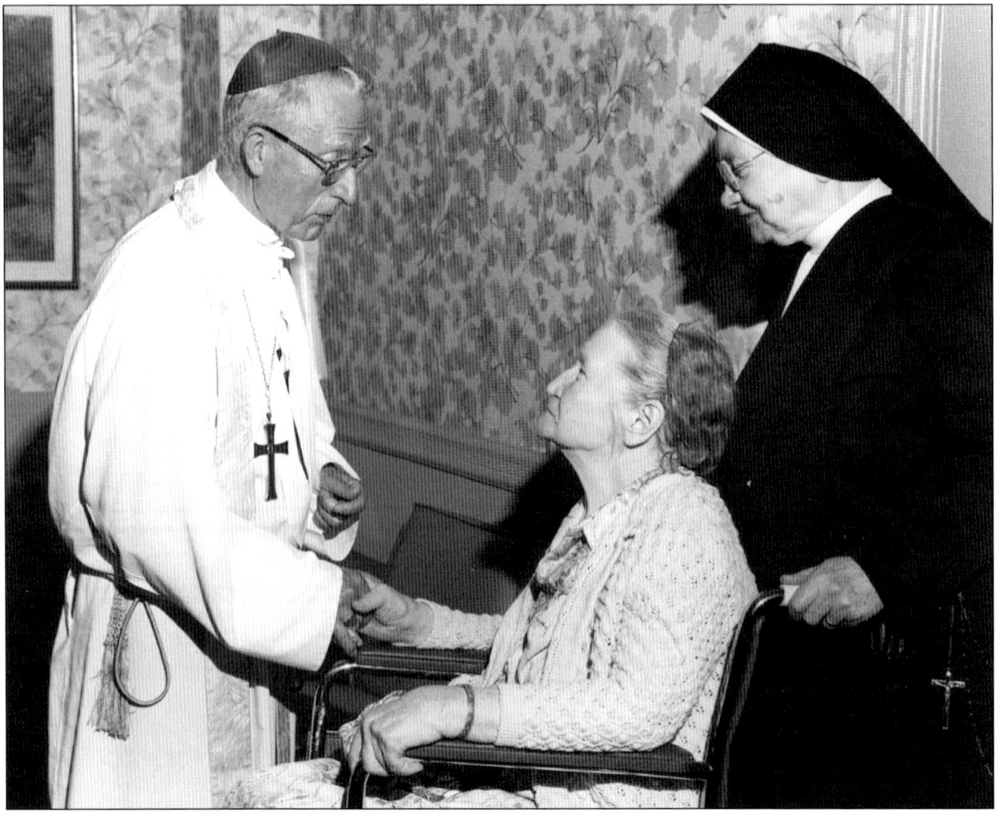

Mother Marie de Lourdes takes a resident to meet a visiting bishop. Mother Marie was a member of the general council, and also served as superior/administrator in five of the Carmelite Sisters' nursing homes.

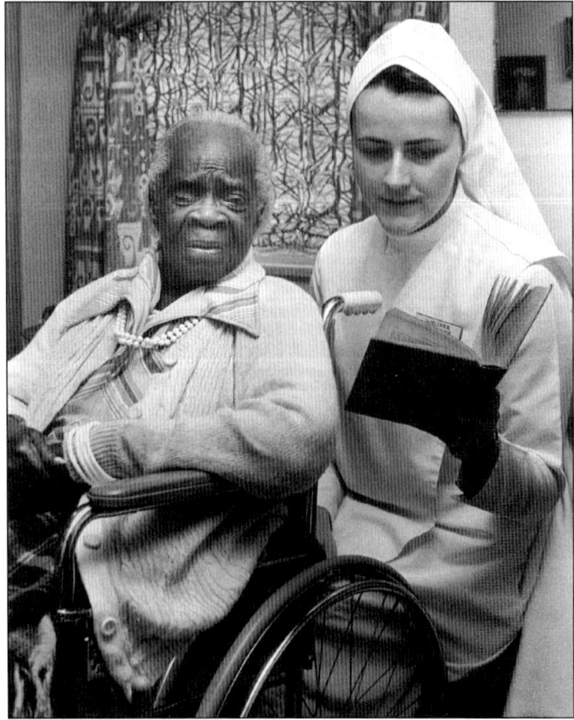

Sr. Helen James reads the Bible to blind resident Mrs. Conroy, who lived to be over 100 years old.

Sr. Mary Robert of the Infant Jesus, administrator of Mary Manning Walsh Home in New York City, gives First Lady Nancy Reagan a tour of the facility.

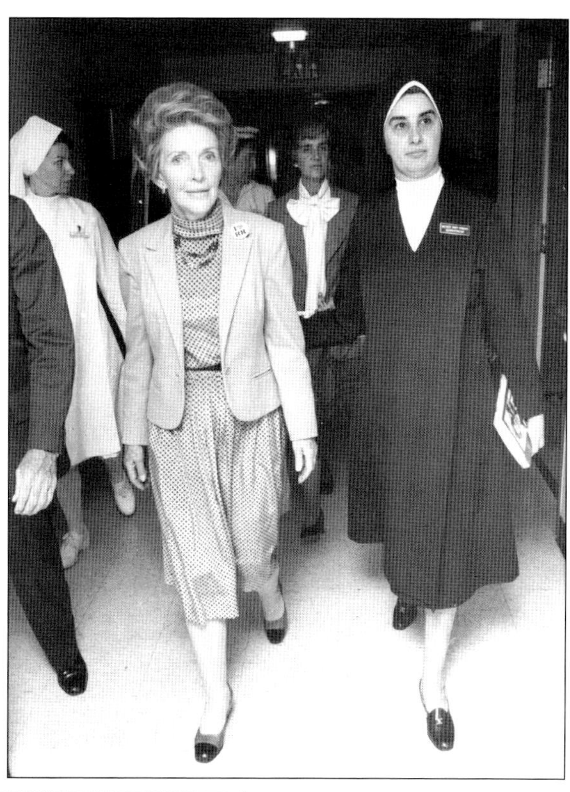

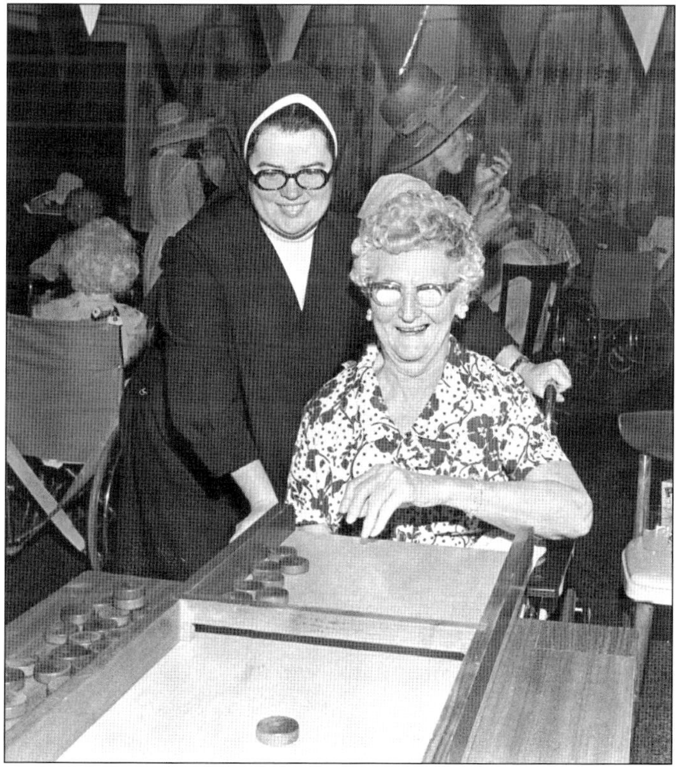

Sr. Margaret Patrick Marie enjoys a chair shuffleboard game with a resident.

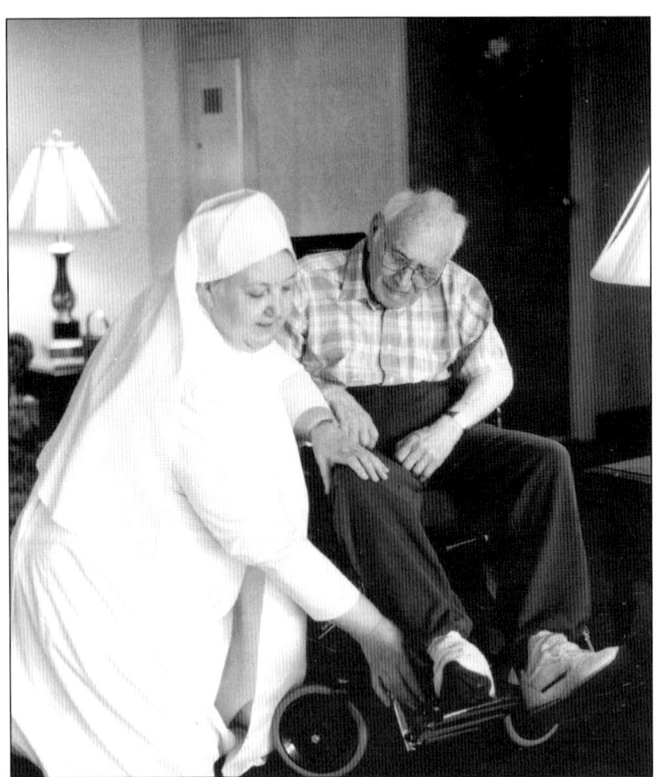

Sr. Carmel Cecilia adjusts the footrest of a resident at Mary Manning Walsh Home.

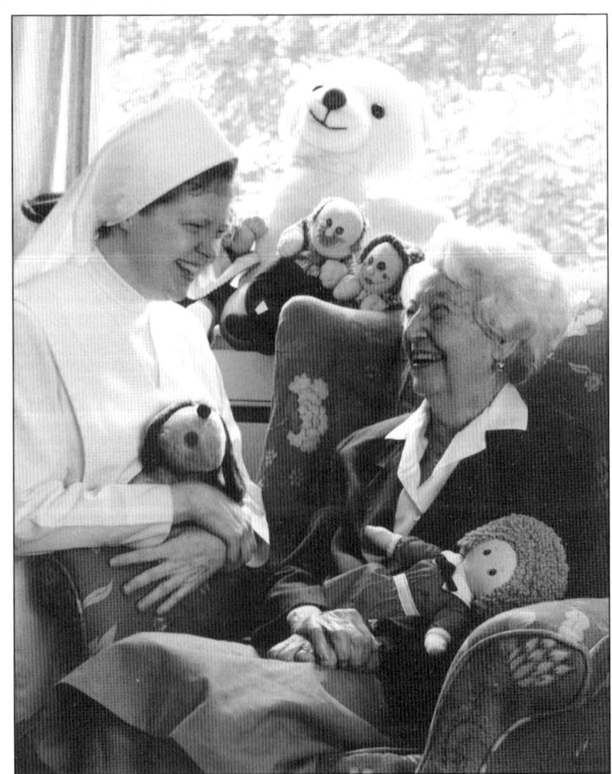

Sr. Raphael Peregrine shares a laugh with a resident at St. Patrick's Residence in Naperville, Illinois. She serves in the Admissions Department.

Sr. Grace Edward takes the blood pressure of a resident. In her later years, she served in Pastoral Ministry at Garvey Manor in Hollidaysburg, Pennsylvania.

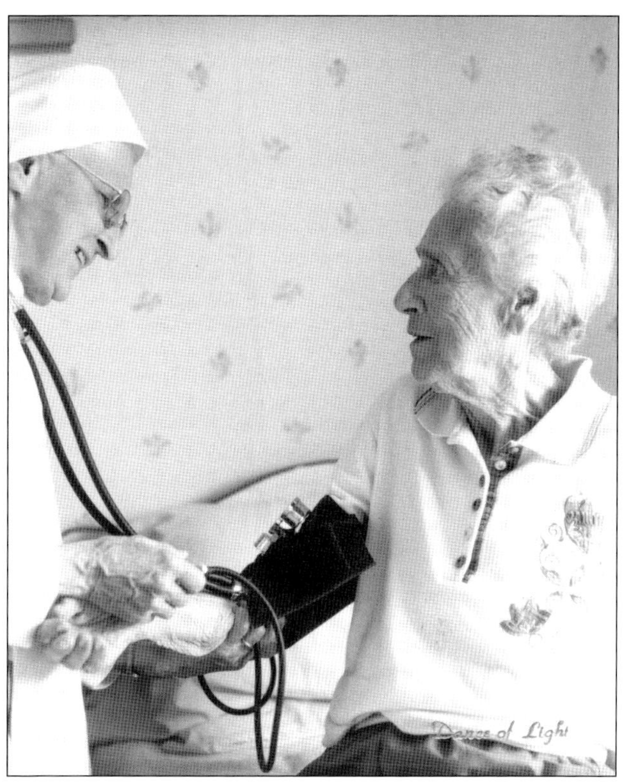

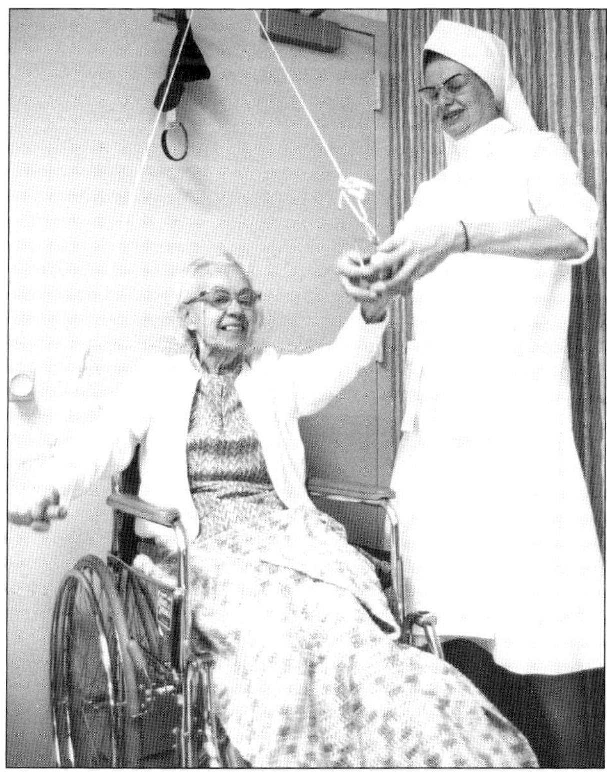

Sr. Charles of St. Joseph works with a resident in occupational therapy to increase her mobility.

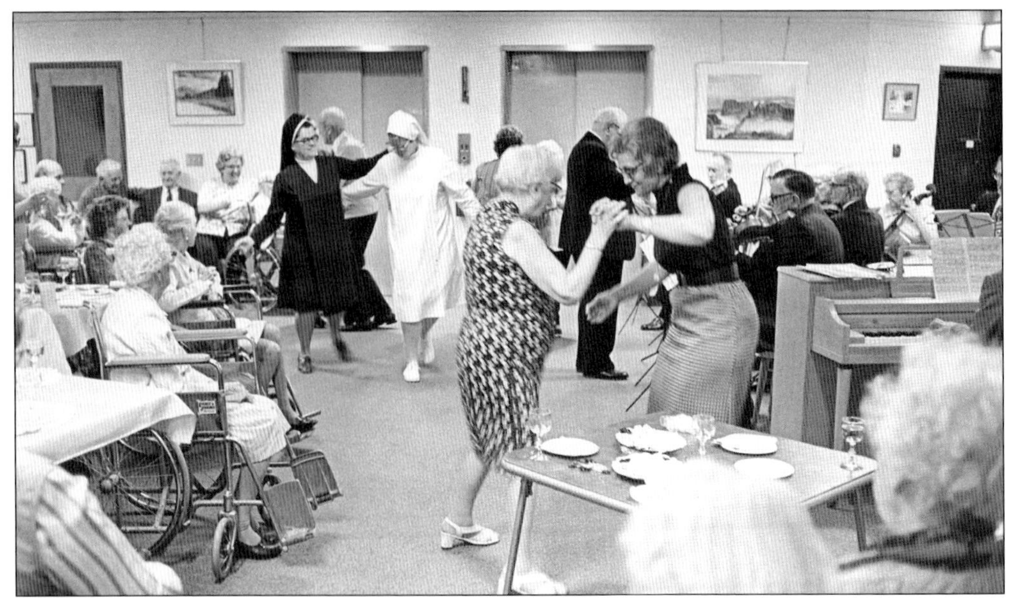

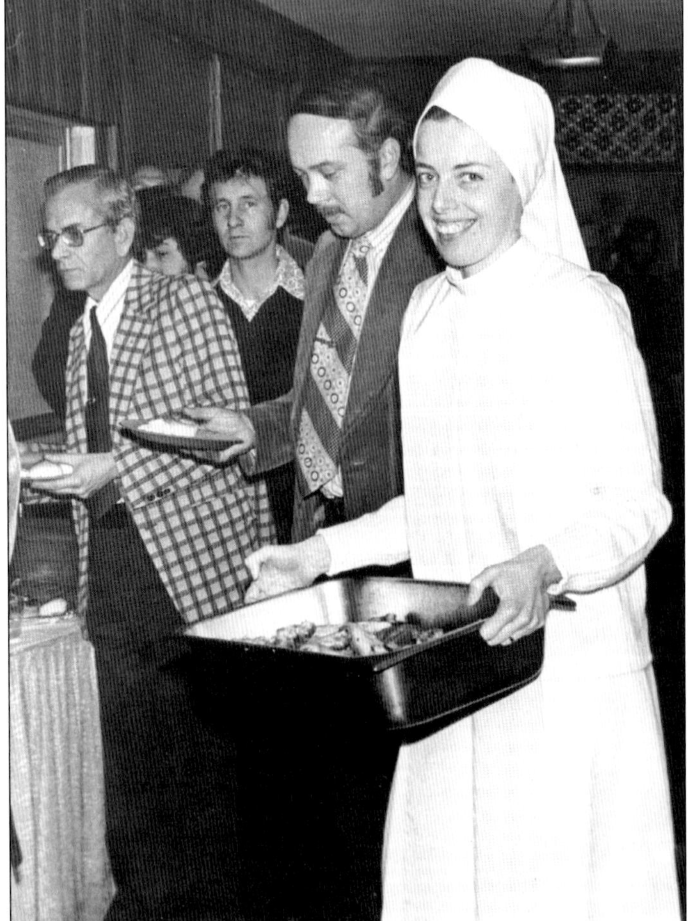

Sr. Margaret Patrick Marie and another sister are dancing to entertain the residents, who so enjoy watching.

Sr. Theresa Cave is seen here carrying food from the kitchen to serve staff at a staff appreciation event. The sisters hold staff appreciation events at all the facilities they sponsor and/or staff.

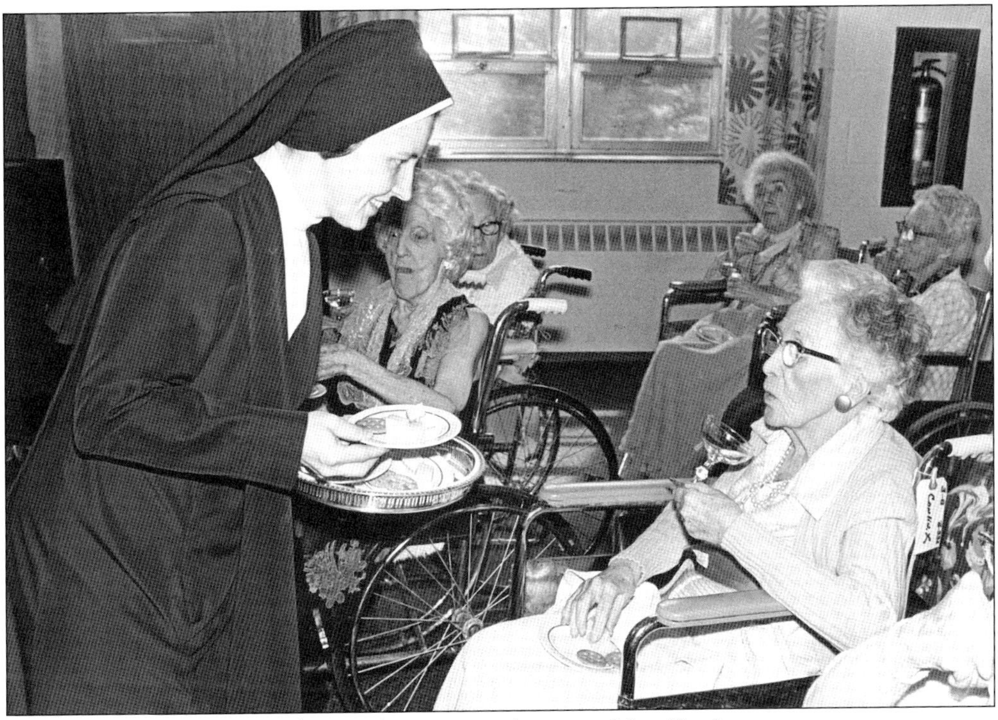

Sr. Kathleen Ann of the Holy Angels serves residents at a New Year's party.

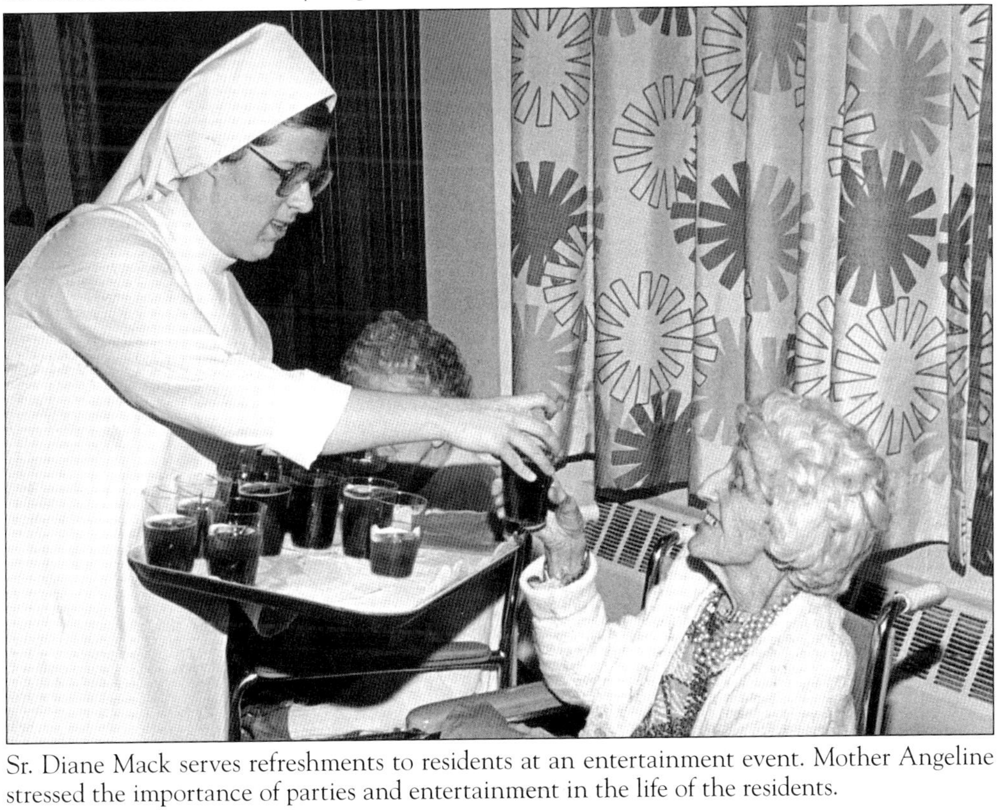

Sr. Diane Mack serves refreshments to residents at an entertainment event. Mother Angeline stressed the importance of parties and entertainment in the life of the residents.

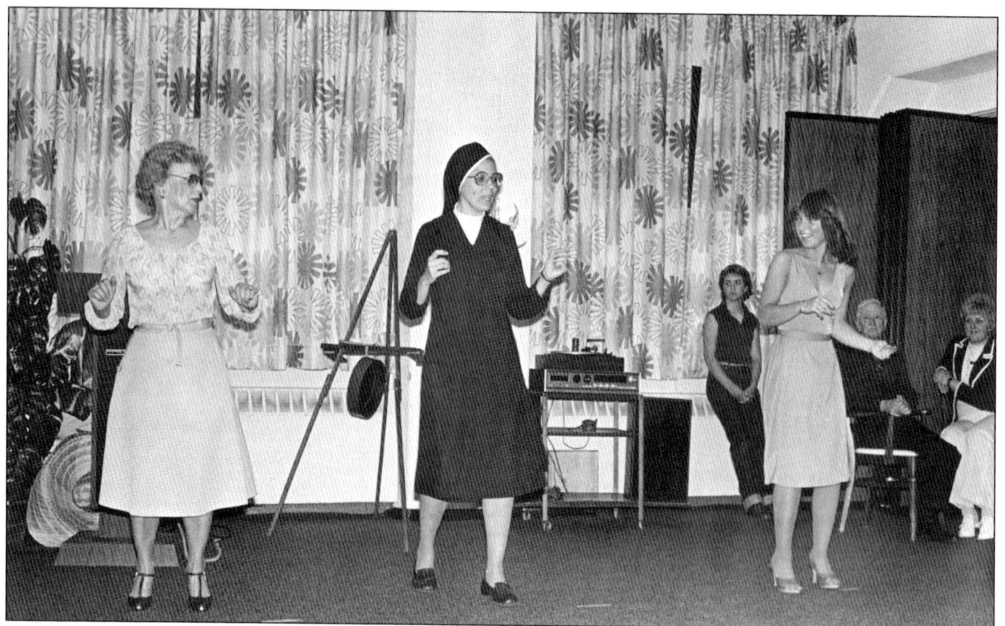

Sr. Madeline Angeline line dances with staff to the delight of the residents. Sisters use their gifts to brighten the lives of the residents and staff.

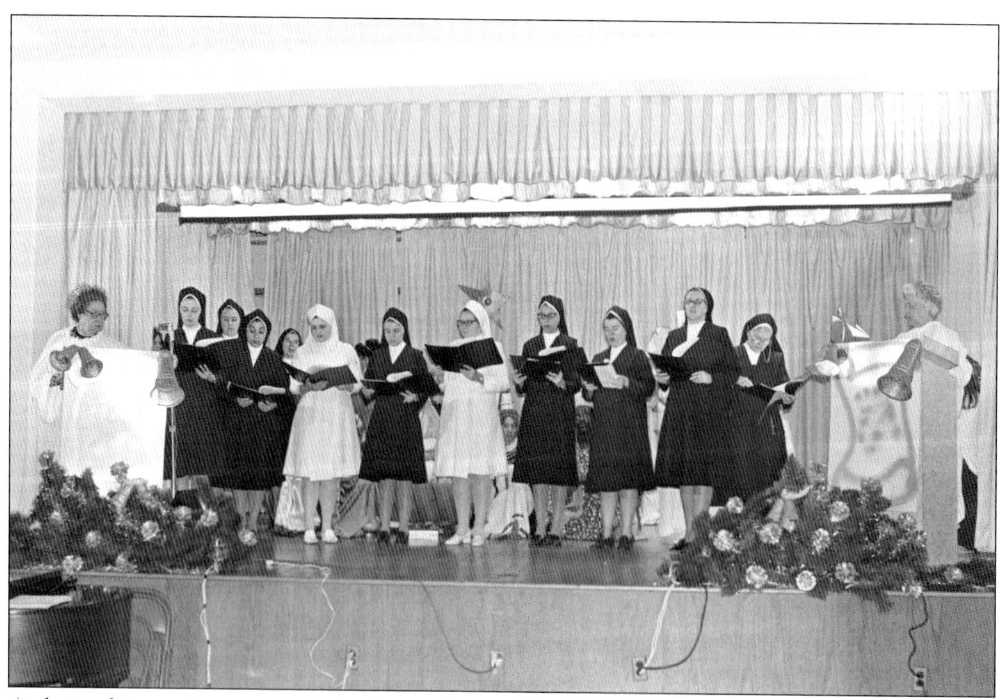

A choir of sisters sings to entertain the residents of St. Joseph's Manor in Trumbull, Connecticut.

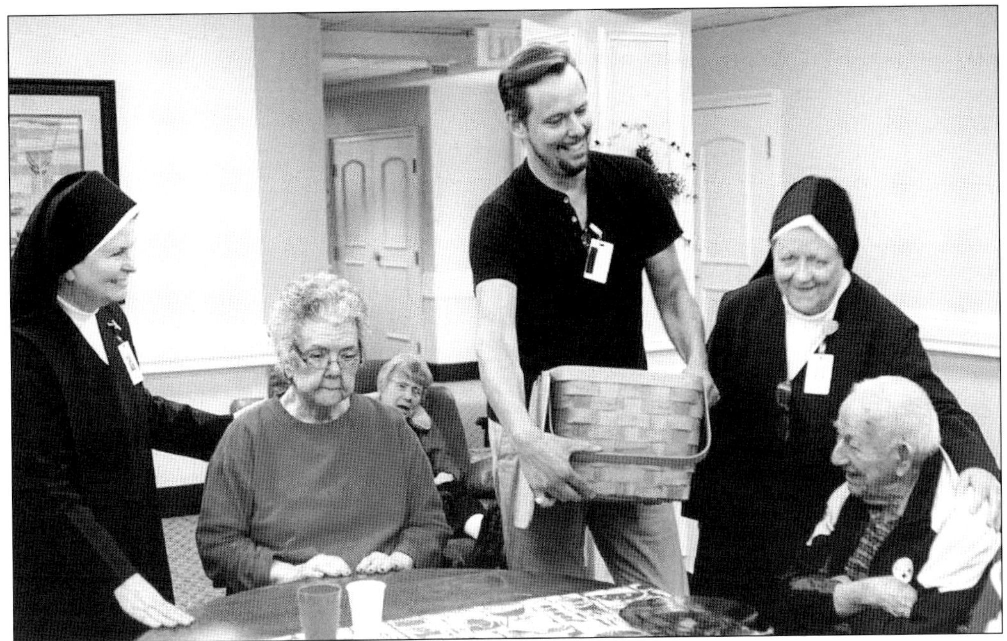

Sr. Maureen Paul Angeline and Sr. Winifred Angeline supervise as a winning number is drawn in a raffle at Mother Angeline McCrory Manor.

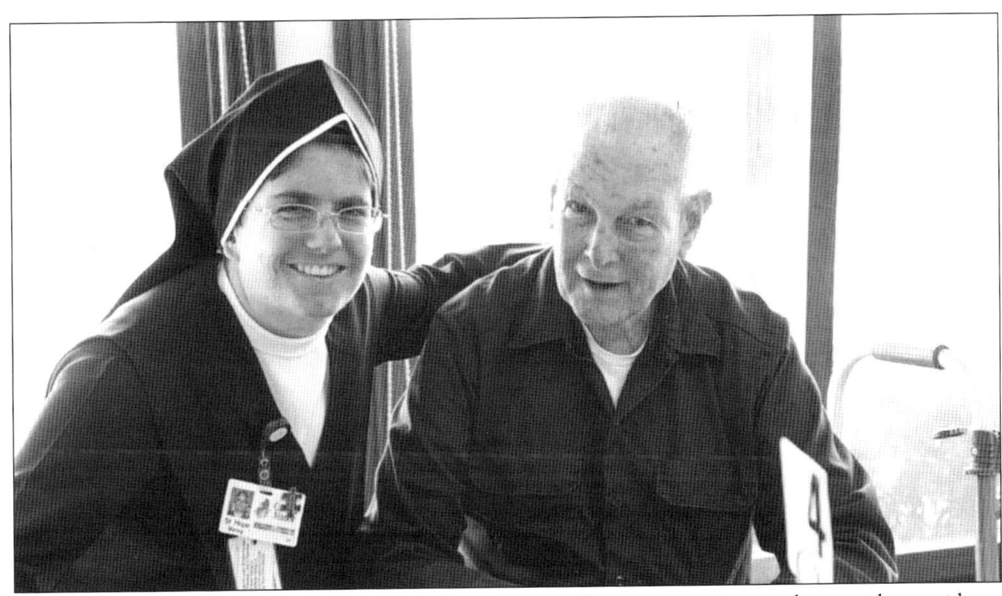

Sr. Hope Therese Angeline, working in the Activities Department, is seen here with a resident.

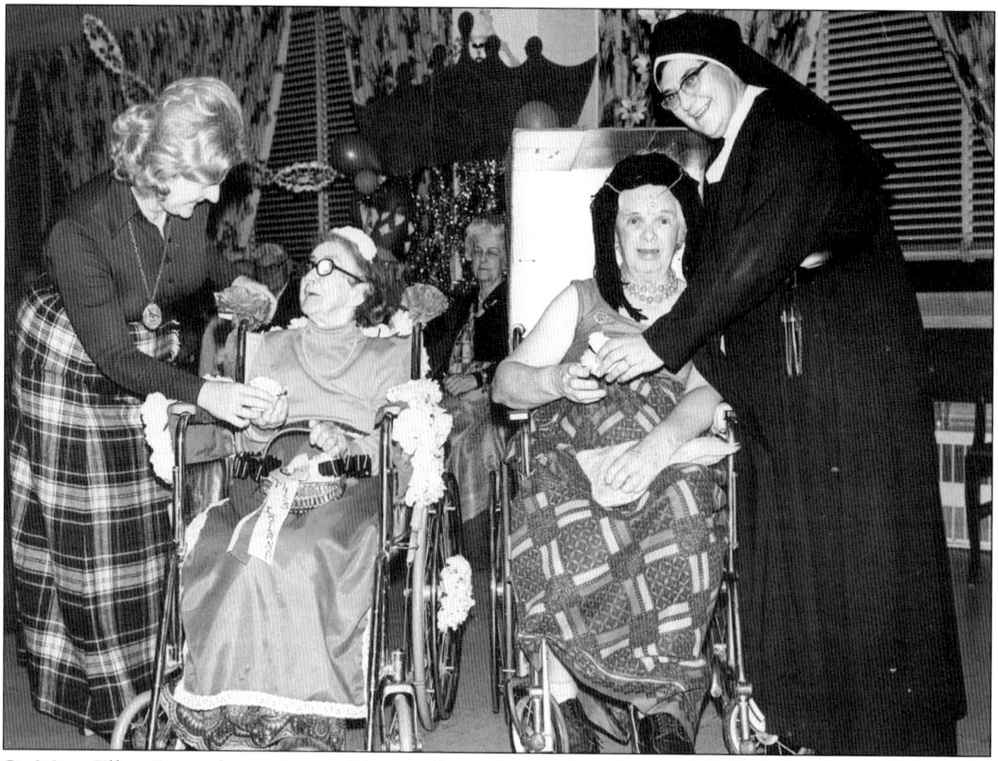

Sr. Mary Ellen Bernadette, along with a staff member and residents, is decked out for a festive event.

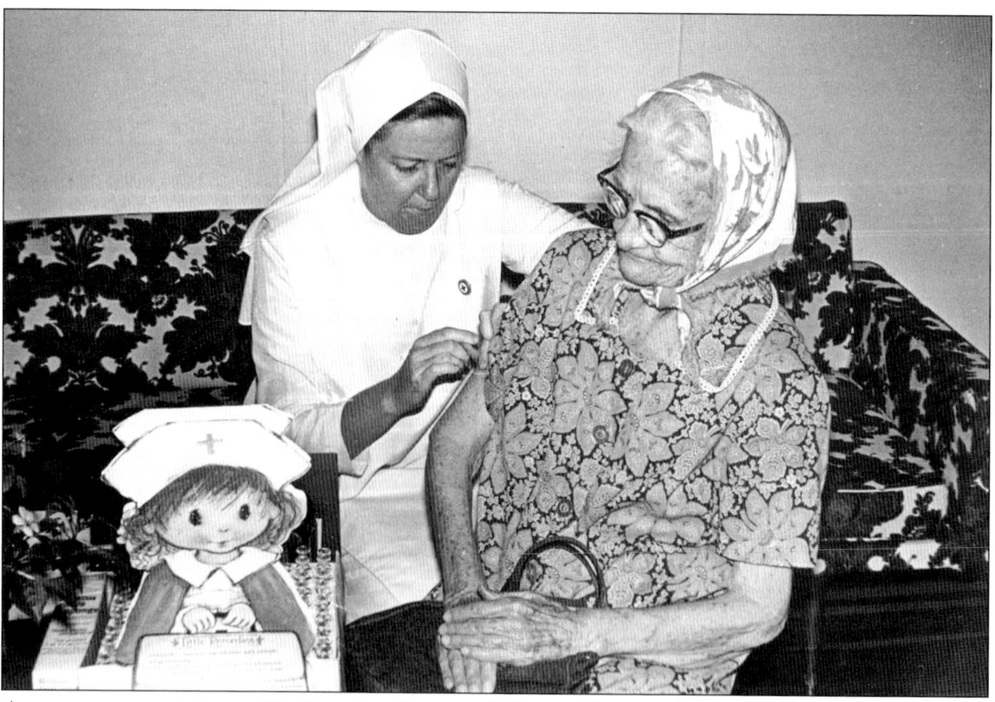

As a nurse practitioner, Sr. Patricia Queen of Carmel knows the importance of preventive maintenance. She is seen here preparing to immunize a resident.

Four

THE CHARISM MULTIPLIES

To further develop the vision of loving care practiced in the facilities, several programs were created to enhance the outreach of the congregation. The Carmelette program involved teenage girls in the sisters' work of caring for the elderly. Many facilities ran a Carmelette program; after 50 hours of volunteer service, the girls received a Carmelette uniform and a pin. Numerous young girls who had volunteered as Carmelettes entered the congregation.

The Mother Angeline Ministries of Care is a volunteer parish outreach program that promotes the ideals of Mother Angeline. Taught by the Carmelite Sisters, this on-site program focuses on bringing Christ to the homebound and the sick of the parish community. Outreach volunteers are trained to mirror Mother Angeline's spirit of kindness, joy, and prayer; they allow each person they visit to feel the compassion and love of Christ in a deeply personal way.

The SALT (Serving Aged Lovingly Today) Carmelite Missionaries program invites young women aged 18-40 to experience the mission and vocation of the Carmelite Sisters for the Aged and Infirm. Over the course of seven days, the participants learn about the mission of Mother Angeline and strengthen their faith through service to the elderly, prayer, conferences, discussions, and days of reflection. SALT participants join residents in their daily activities and play games, sit, talk, and pray with them. The program is hosted at one of the nursing homes or assisted living facilities of the Carmelite Sisters. This gives the young women an opportunity to discover the joy the sisters find in their ministry and in their religious life.

The Avila Institute of Gerontology, incorporated in 1988, was initiated by the Carmelite Sisters for the Aged and Infirm to respond to the growing complexity of geriatric health care. As the educational arm of the congregation, the institute offers education, training, and consulting that helps to meet the needs of all long-term care professionals and caregivers, including administrators, nurses, social workers, recreational therapists, dietitians, spiritual caregivers, and other health-care professionals.

Roots of Caring is a leadership program for staff employed at facilities served by the congregation. Education focuses on the mission of the sisters, Catholic health care, and topics of leadership formation.

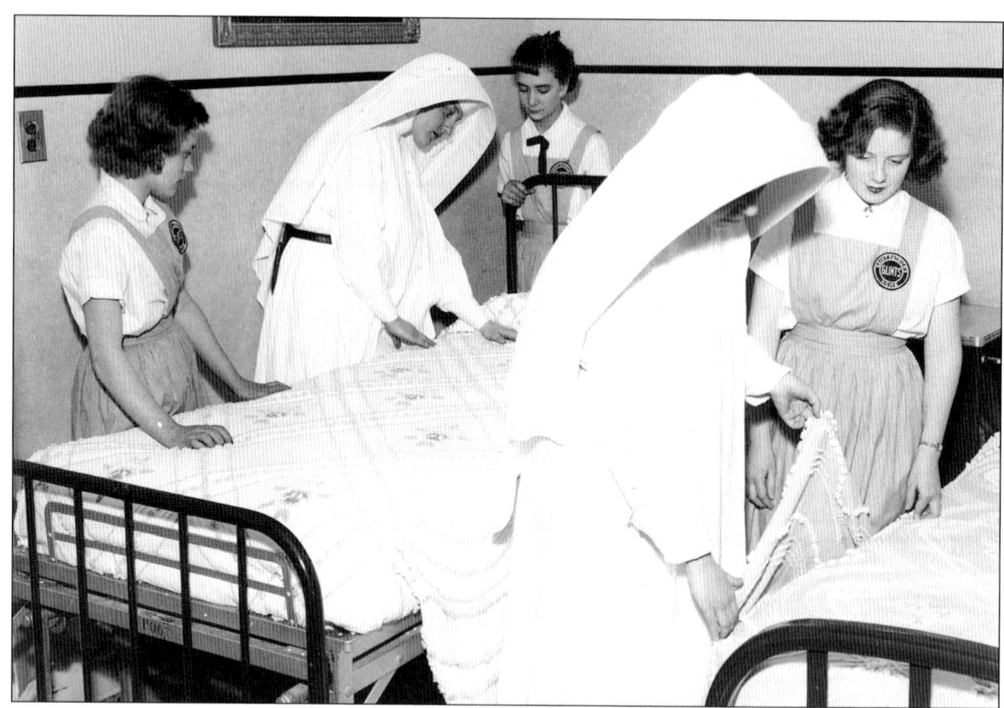

Sisters train Carmelettes on how to make a bed with sheets folded in hospital corners.

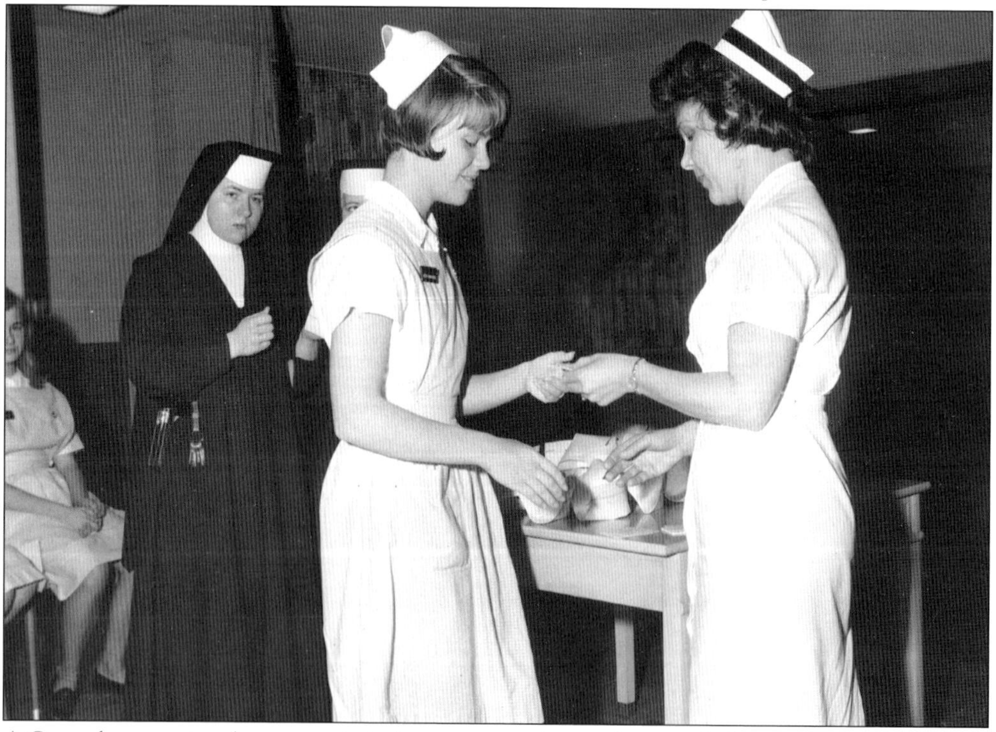

A Carmelette receives her cap and pin from a nurse after performing 50 hours of volunteer service as Sr. Kevin Patricia of the Holy Angels looks on. Each of the facilities that had Carmelette programs had slightly different uniforms for the girls.

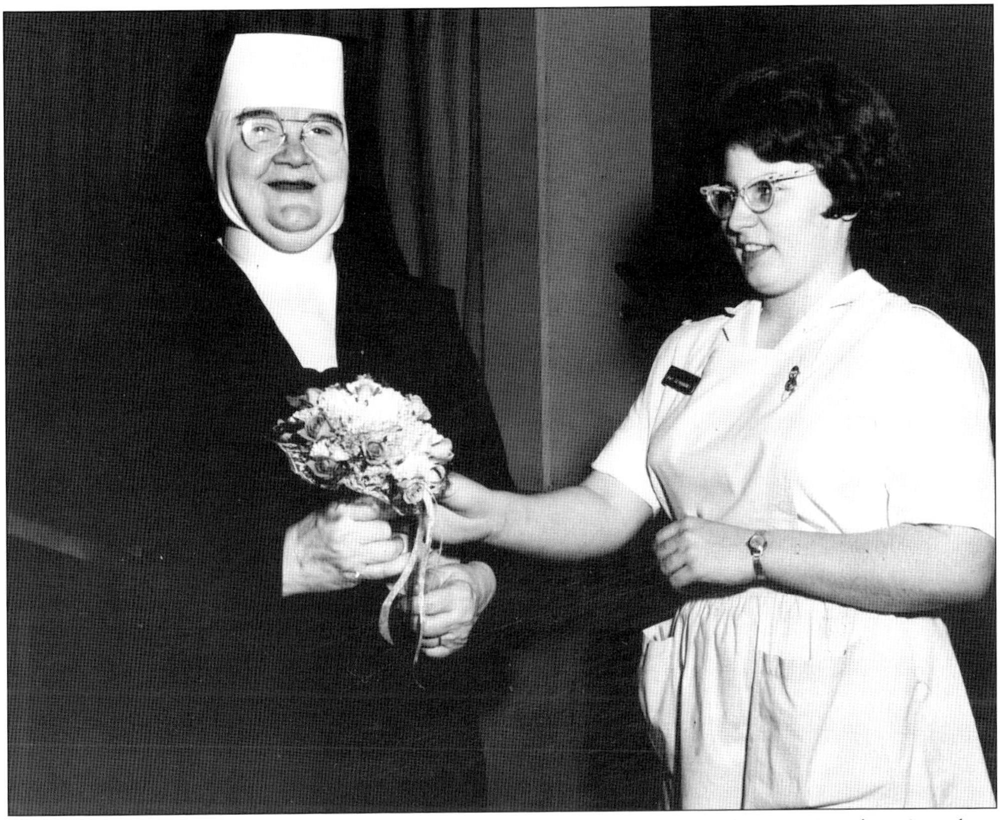

Mother Angeline receives a bouquet of flowers from a Carmelette volunteer. Mother Angeline made the rounds of each of the nursing homes at least yearly and always took the time to visit with the Carmelettes.

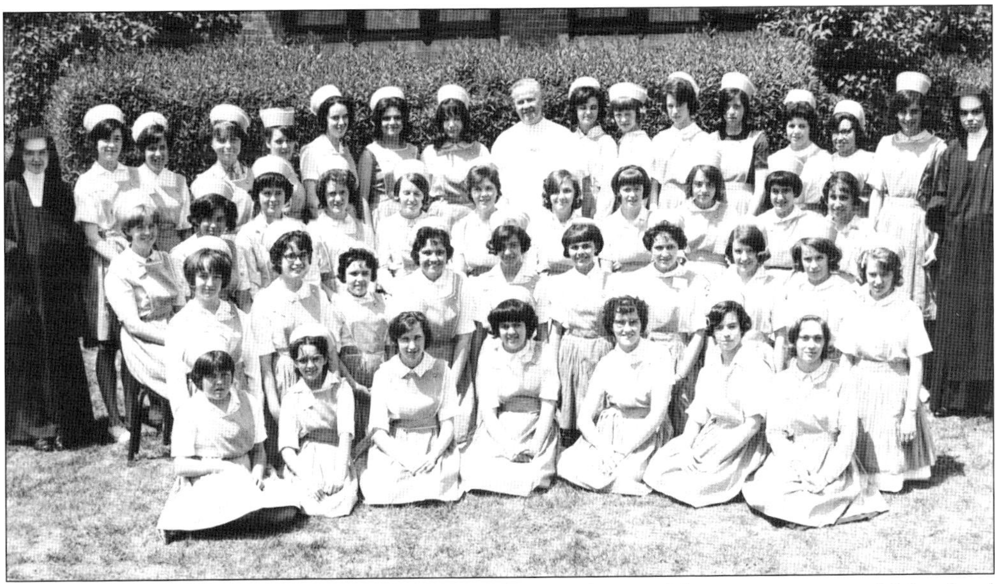

This group photograph of 41 Carmelettes shows the popularity of the program among high school girls at Our Lady's Haven in Fairhaven, Massachusetts.

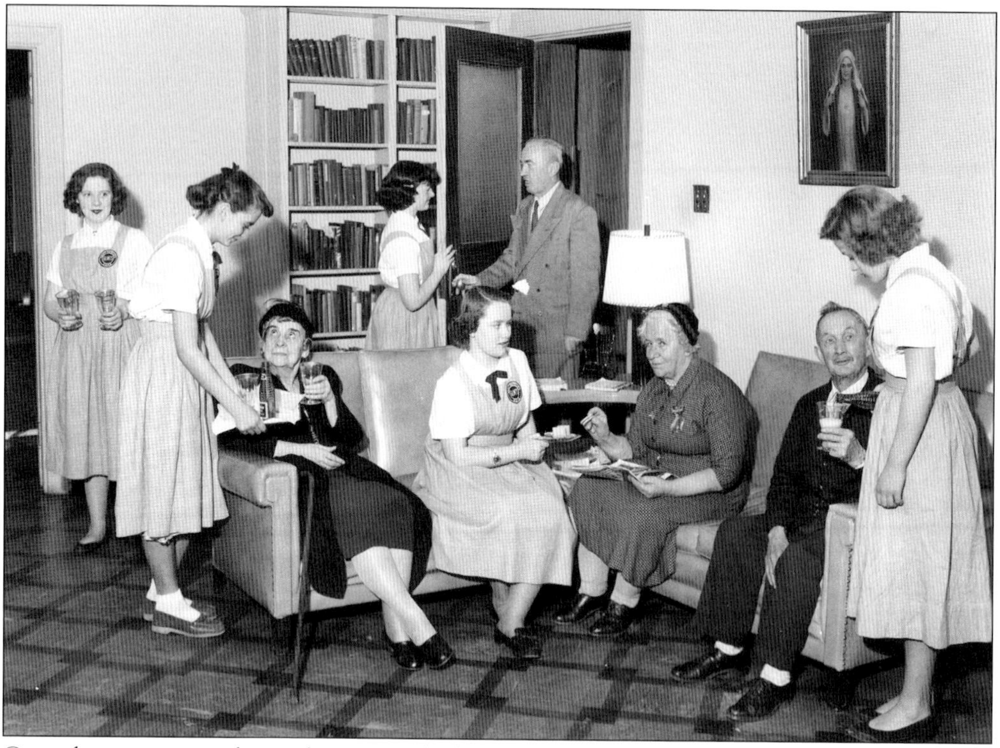

Carmelettes serve residents afternoon refreshments and spend some time visiting with them.

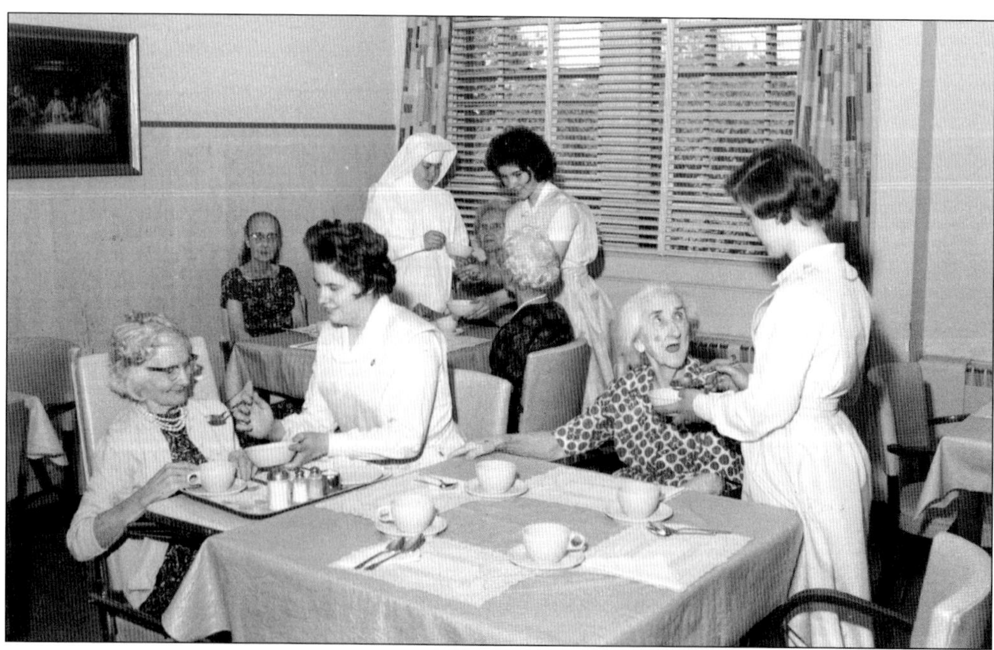

Under the watchful eye of a sister, these Carmelettes are serving the residents a meal or helping them eat their meal.

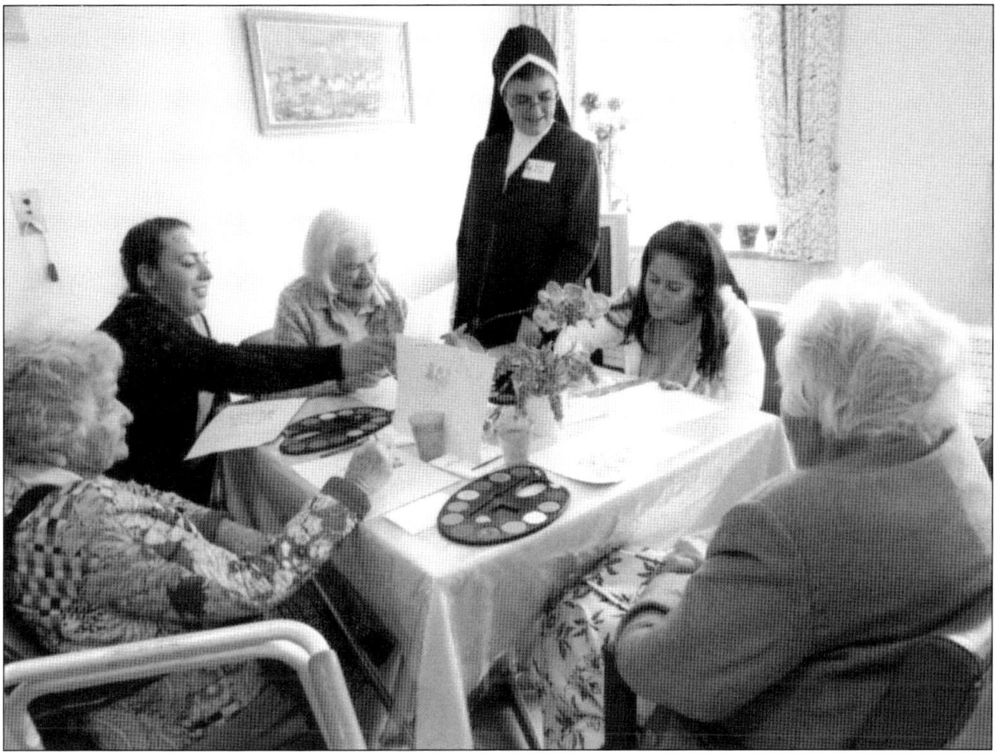

Sr. Mary of Jesus, director of vocations, supervises Kristen Pohl and Kassandra Heflin, SALT missionaries, as they work with residents at Our Lady's Manor nursing home in Dalkey, Ireland.

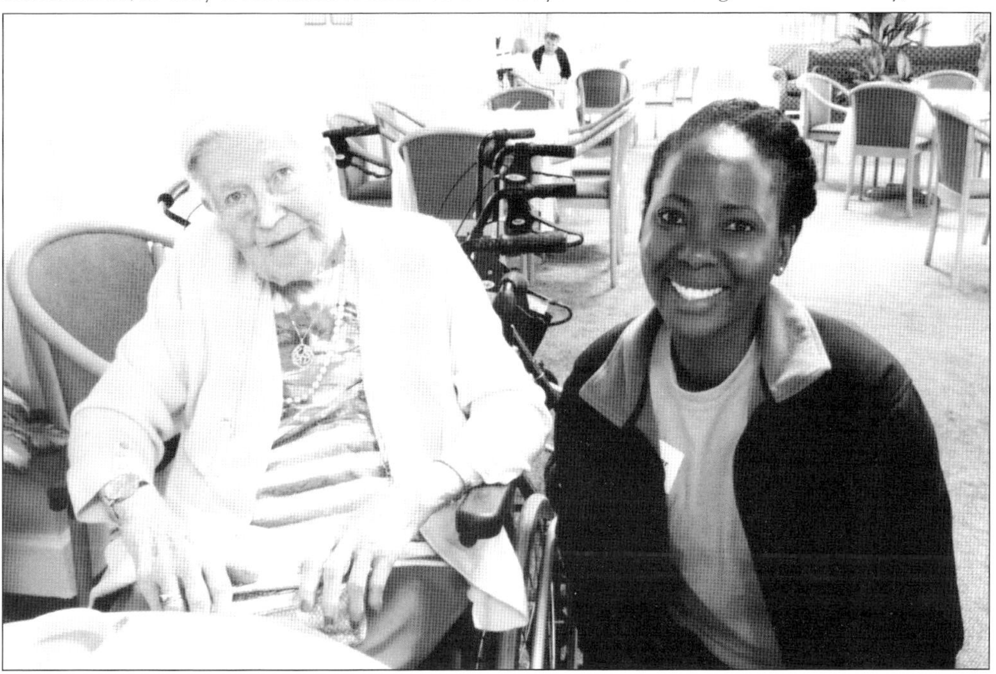

SALT missionary Heather George visits with a resident of Our Lady's Manor during an activities program.

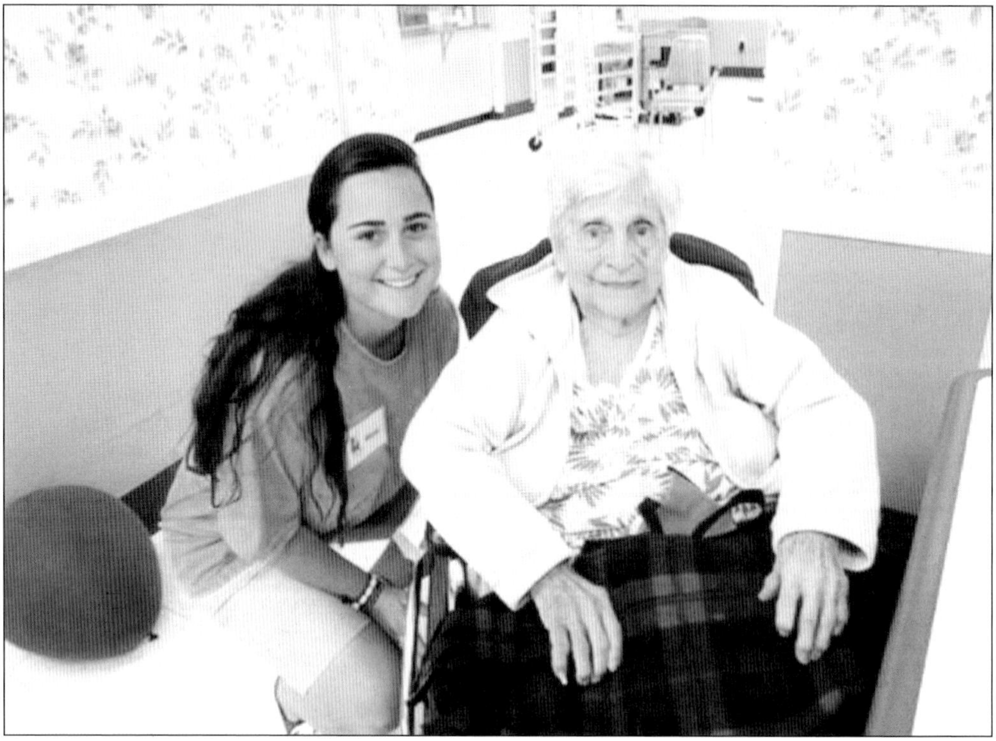

SALT missionary Alyssa DiMaria visits with a resident in the coffee shop of Our Lady's Manor.

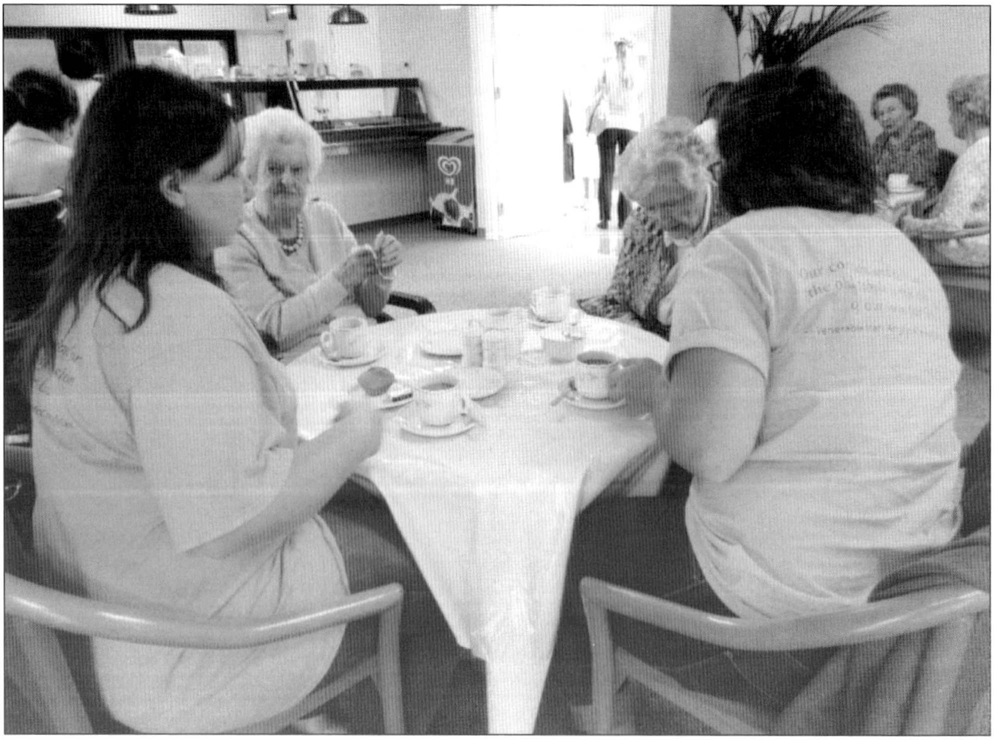

SALT missionaries work one-on-one with two residents at snack time at this table.

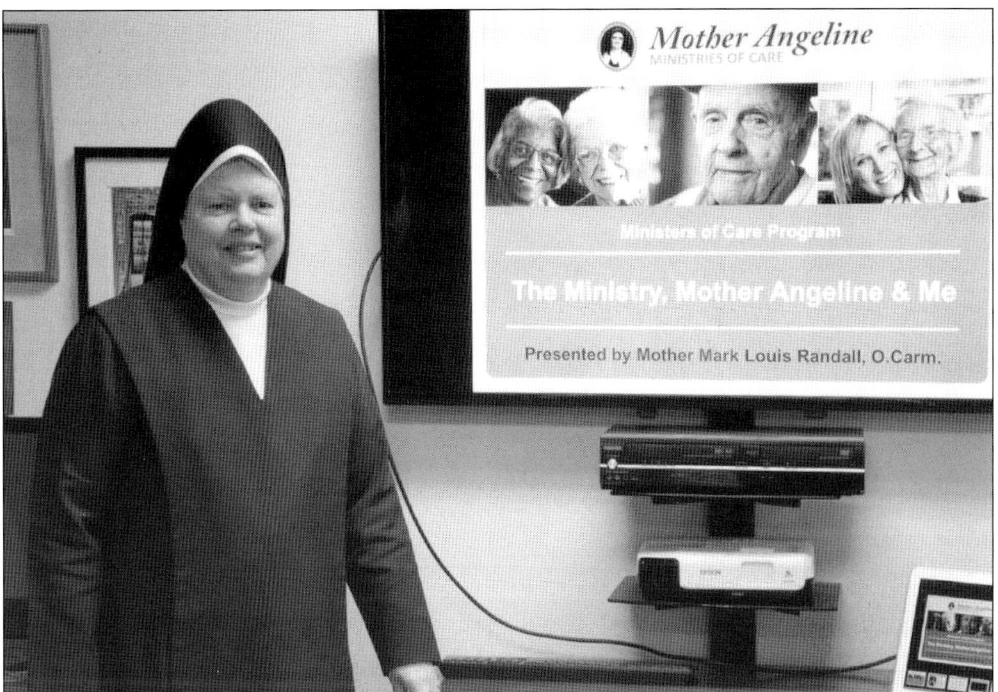

Mother Mark Louis Anne opens a session that is a part of the Mother Angeline Ministries of Care training that the sisters provide to parish ministers to the homebound.

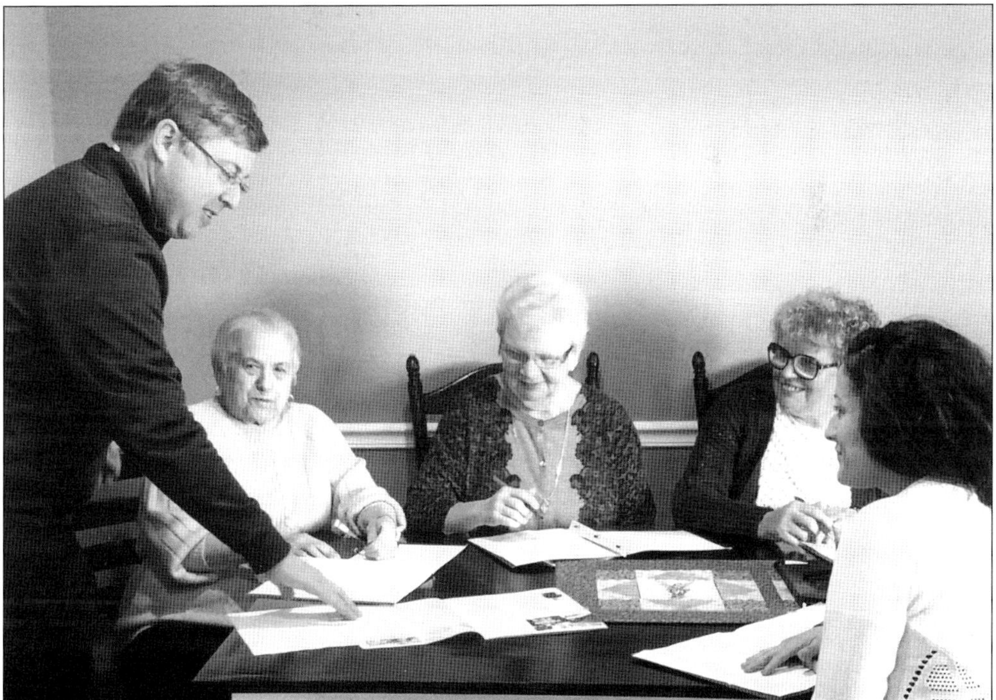

Rev. Andrew Nelson is seen here providing further training to Mother Angeline Ministers of Care in the St. Ignatius of Loyola Parish in Somersworth, New Hampshire.

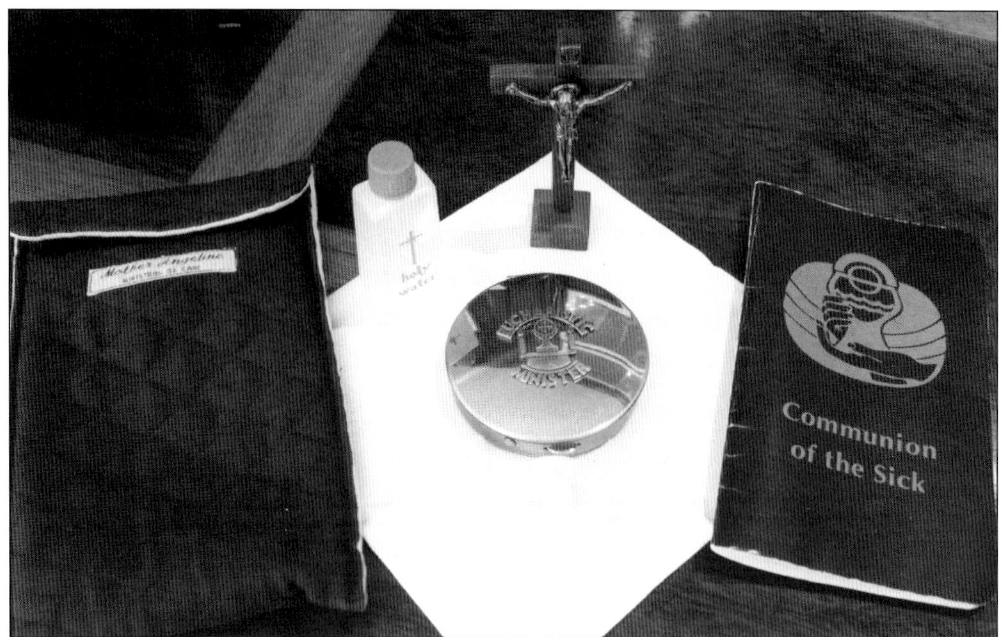

This is the Mother Angeline Ministers of Care kit that is provided to all the commissioned ministers of care. It is comprised of a pyx, a crucifix, a candle, a holy water bottle, a Communion of the Sick booklet, and a white cloth to place the devotional objects on.

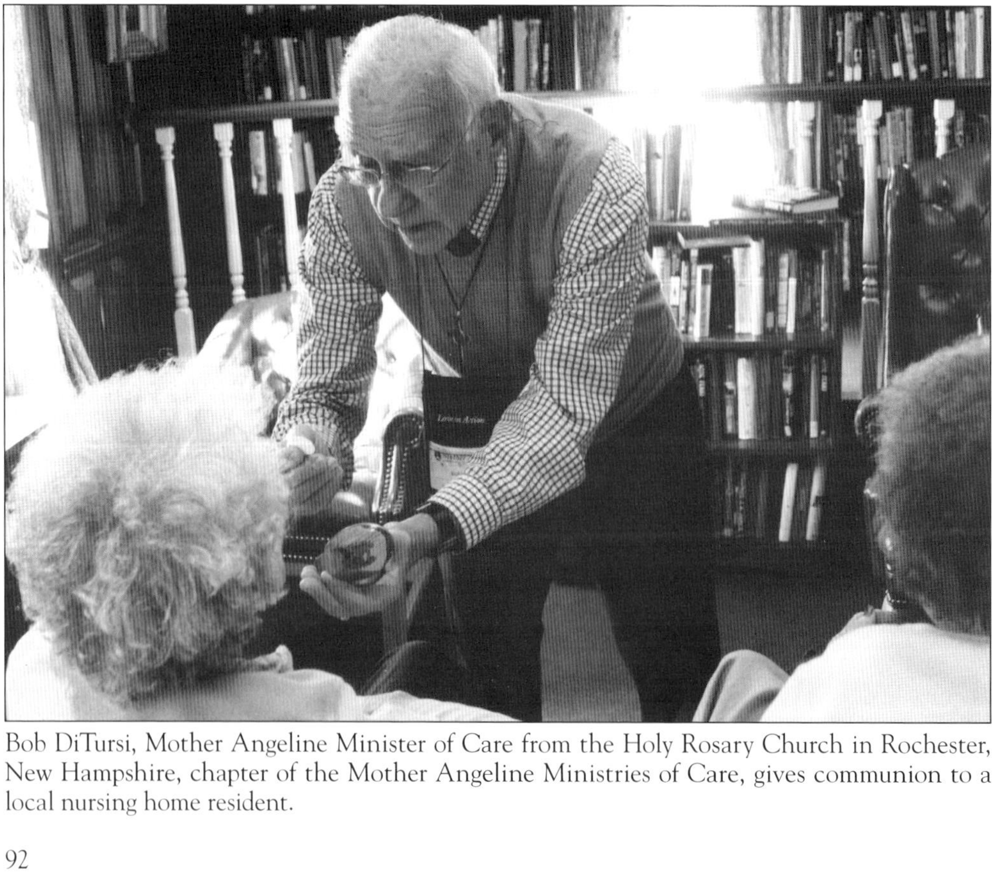

Bob DiTursi, Mother Angeline Minister of Care from the Holy Rosary Church in Rochester, New Hampshire, chapter of the Mother Angeline Ministries of Care, gives communion to a local nursing home resident.

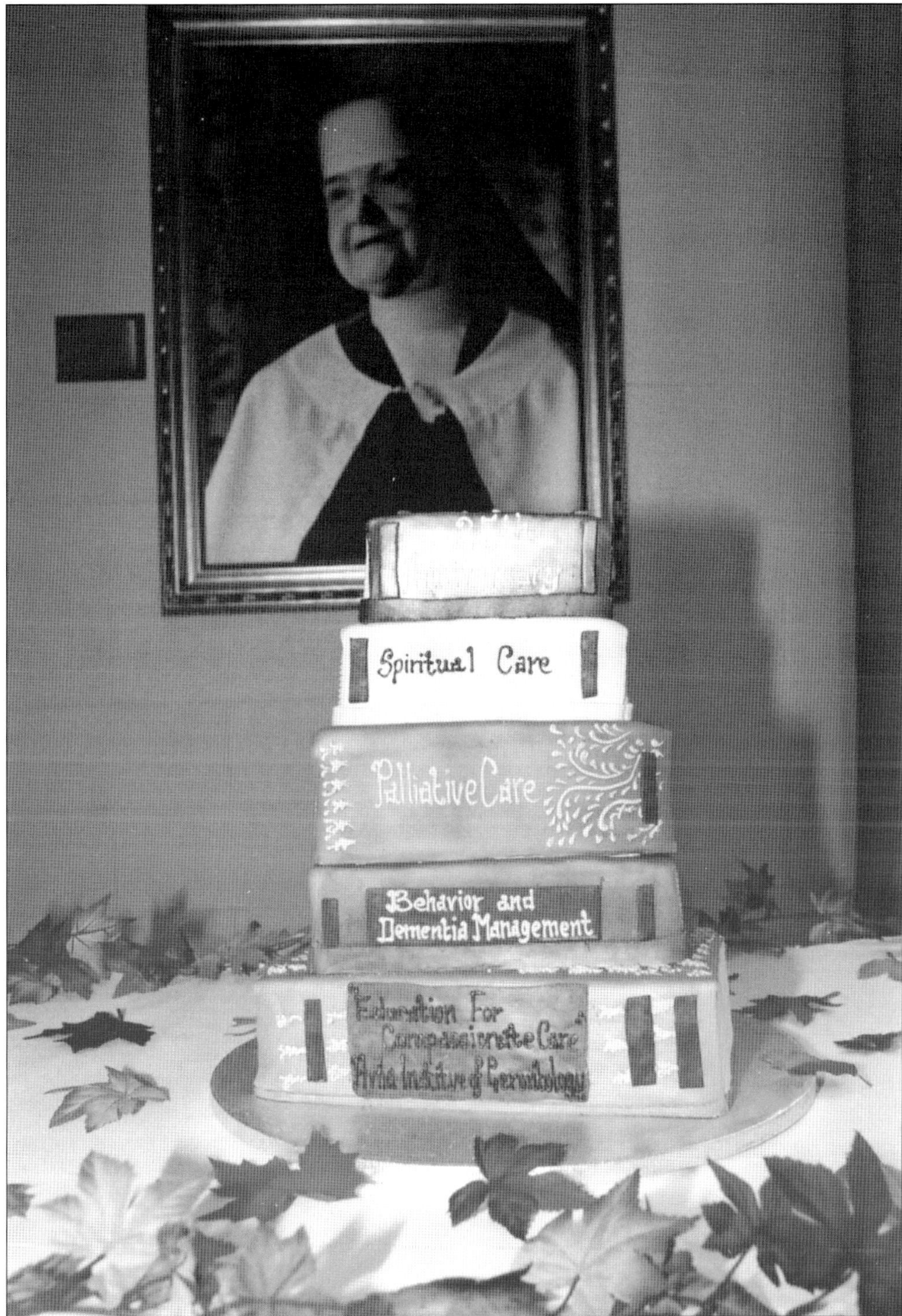

The Avila Institute of Gerontology, the educational arm of the Carmelite Sisters for the Aged and Infirm, celebrated its 25th anniversary in 2013. This anniversary cake with tiers represented the various programs developed by the institute.

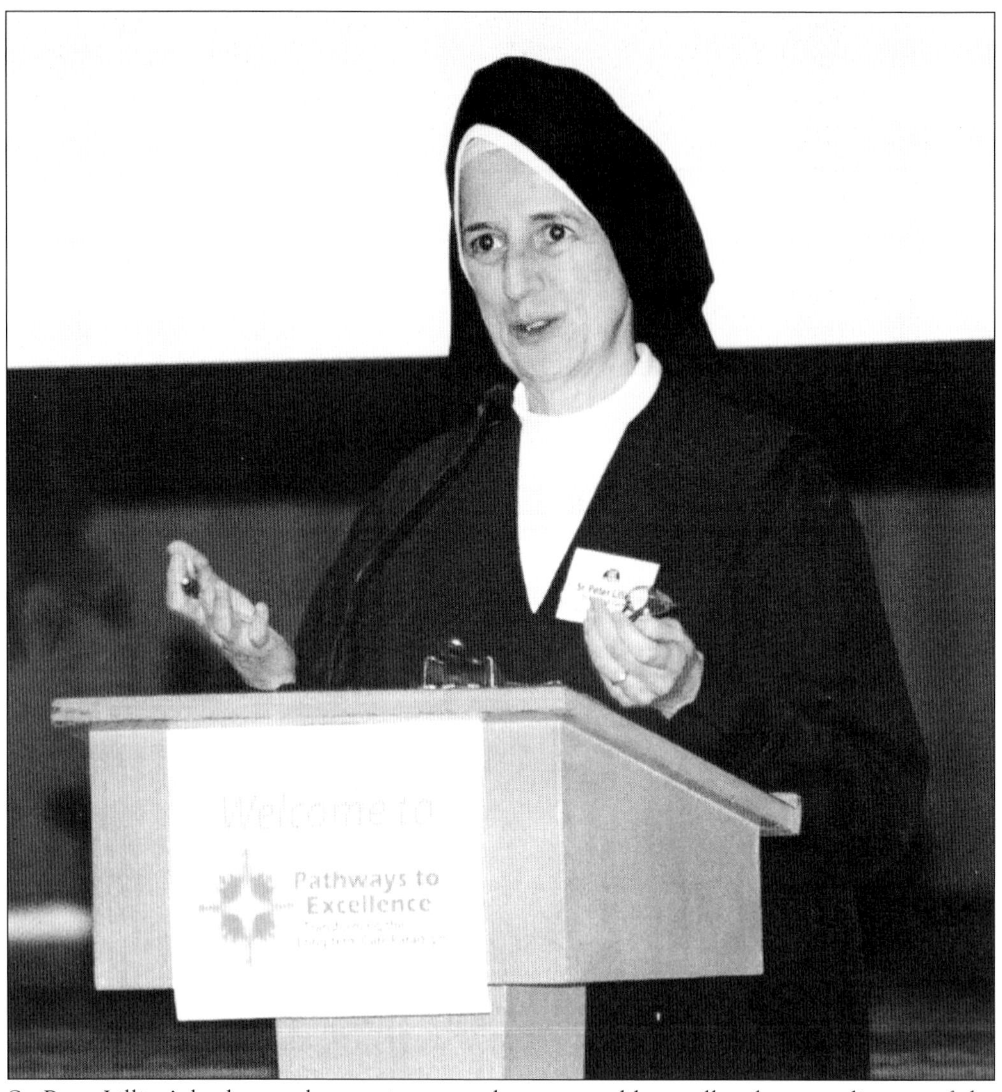

Sr. Peter Lillian's background as a science teacher prepared her well to become director of the Avila Institute. Here, she lectures to attendees in a seminar centered on "Pathways to Excellence."

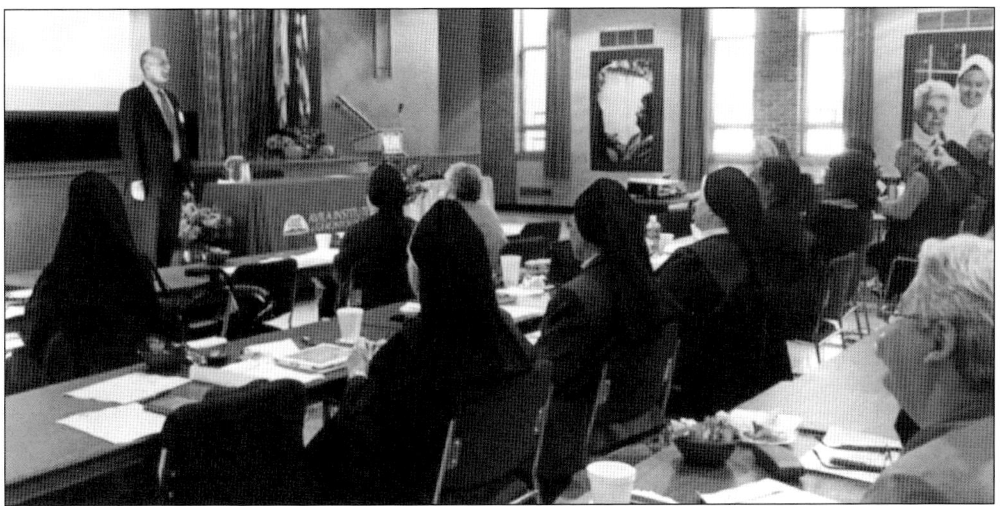

The Avila Institute of Gerontology sponsors multiple webinars and a yearly seminar in October for nursing home administrators and staff. It is held in Carmel Hall, an all-purpose room located on the motherhouse grounds. This photograph shows one of the speakers as he addresses seminar attendees.

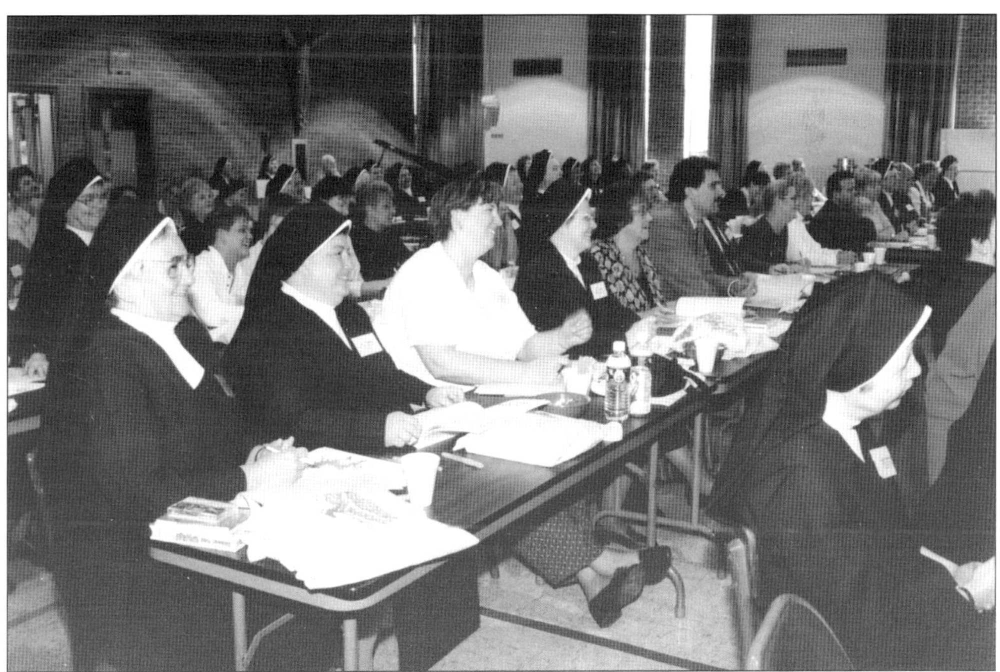

Attendees at one of the seminars share a laugh with the speaker.

Role of Participants

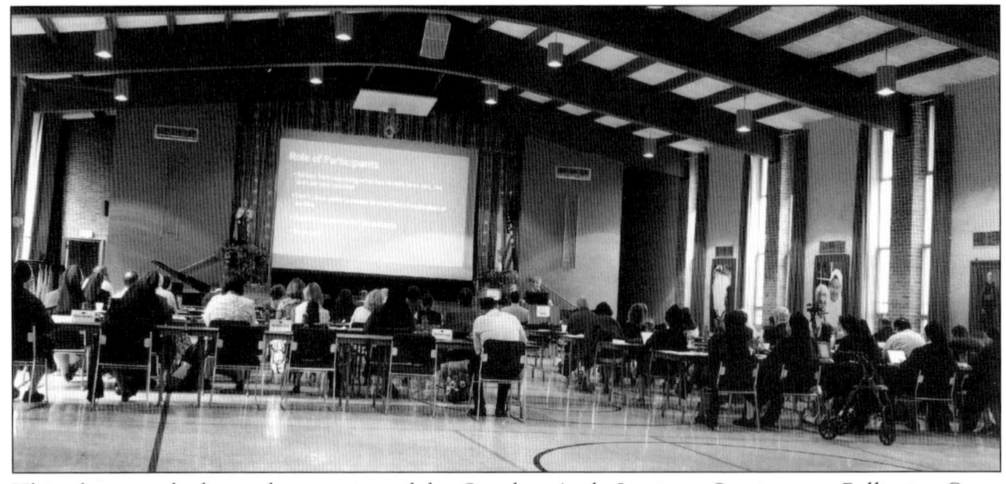

This photograph shows the opening of the October Avila Institute Seminar on Palliative Care. The sisters always open seminars with a call to prayer.

PALLIATIVE CARE – DEFINITION 1
"Palliative care seeks to prevent, relieve, reduce or soothe the

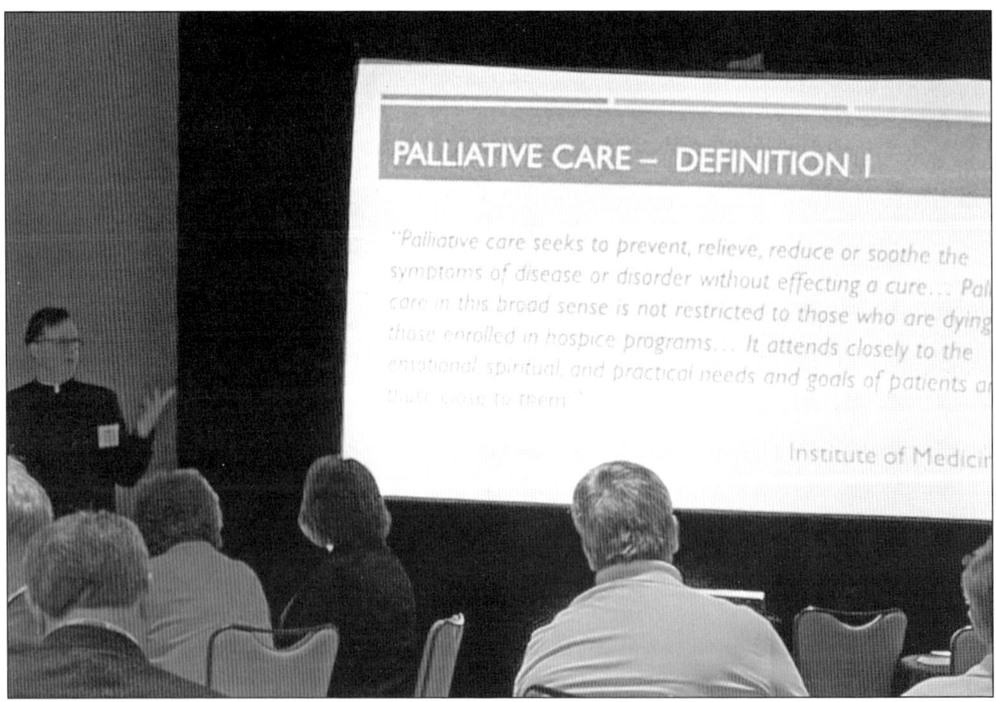

Rev. Dr. Myles Sheehan presented on "Palliative Sedation: Cautions, Concerns, and Indications" as visiting faculty for the Avila Institute of Gerontology.

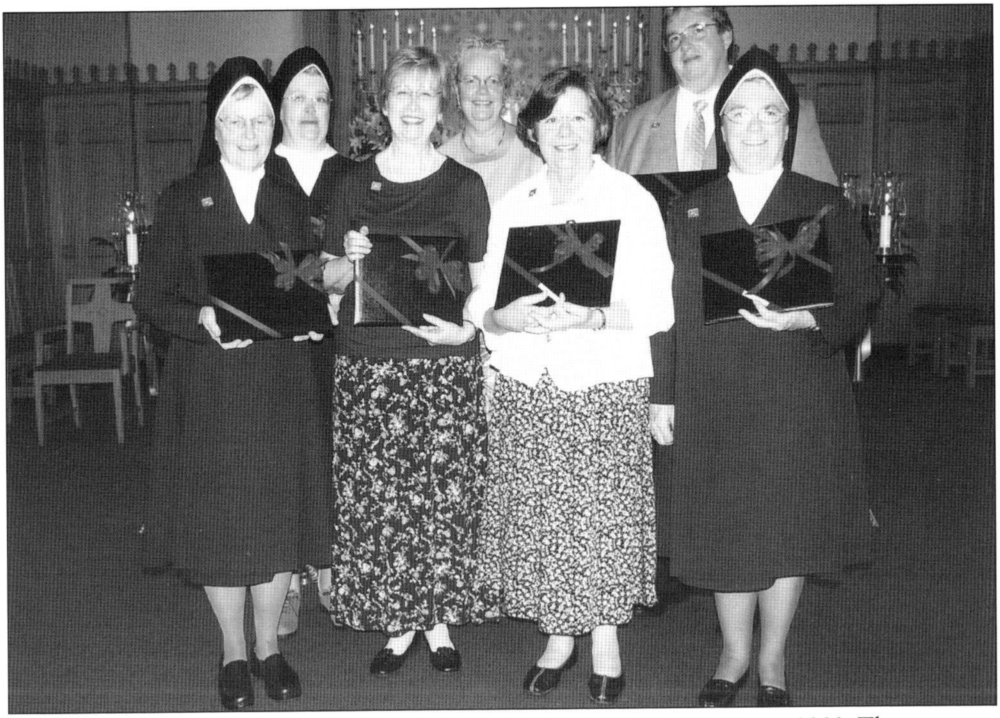

Pictured here are the graduates of the Geriatric Spiritual Care program in 2009. The sisters in the photograph are Sr. Shawn Bernadette (far left), Sr. Patricia Eileen (second from left), and Sr. Alice Webster (far right).

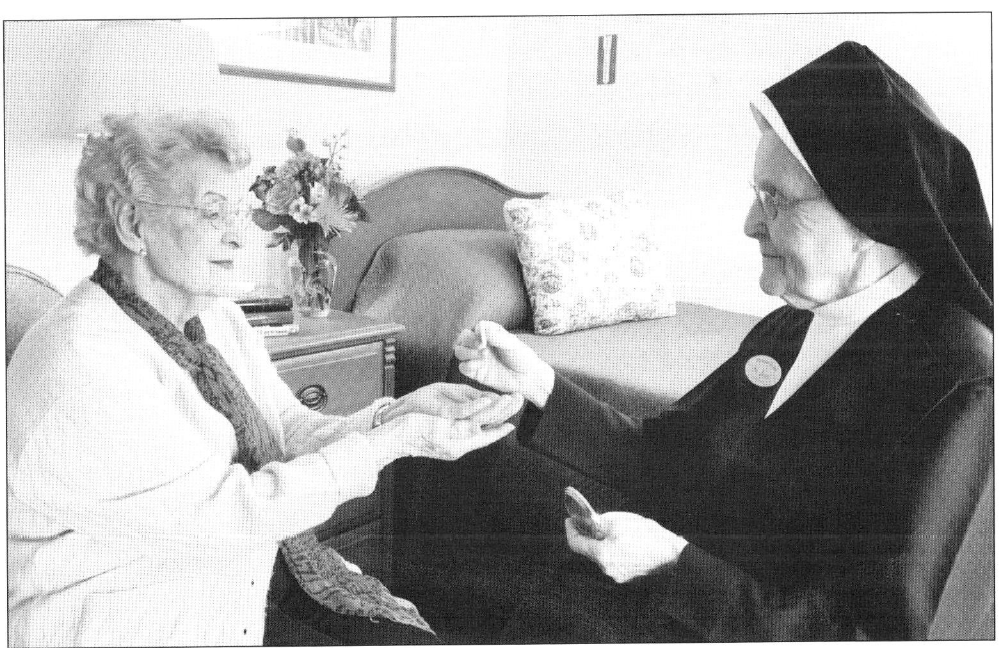

Sr. Joan Mary Lewis, pastoral care minister, brings communion to Jacqueline Van Voorhis in her room at Teresian House in Albany, New York.

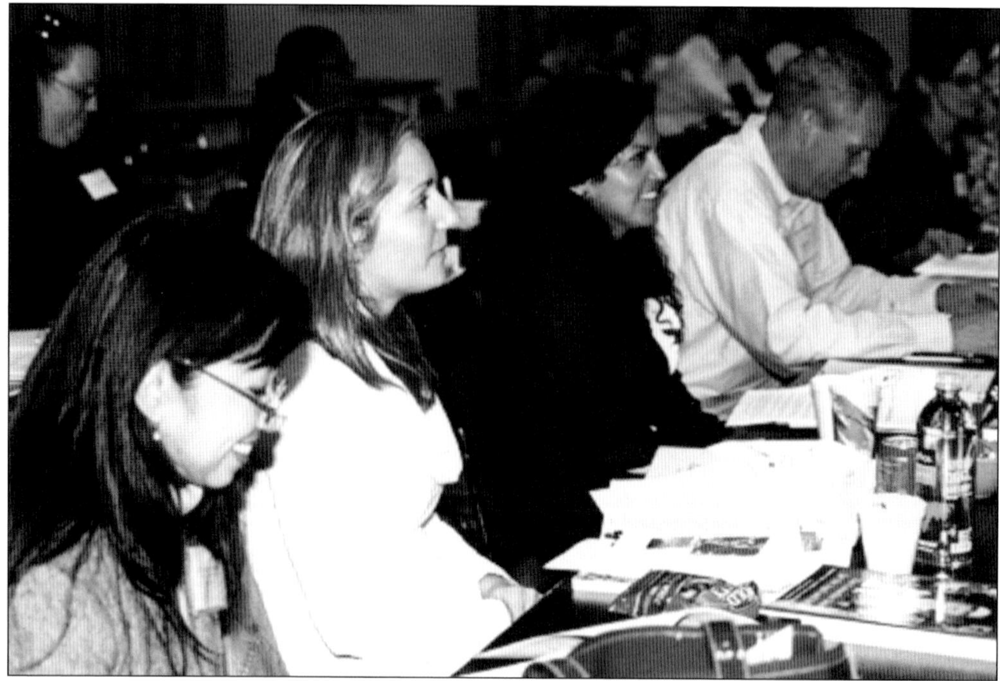

Roots of Caring trainees, all employees of the Carmelite care facilities, undergo a formation that is divided into three modules: Mission, Catholic Healthcare, and Management, which take place over a period of 18 months. The participants need to complete classes and take part in two conference calls to go over an assignment that takes place in between modules. They also have a final project; everything is graded.

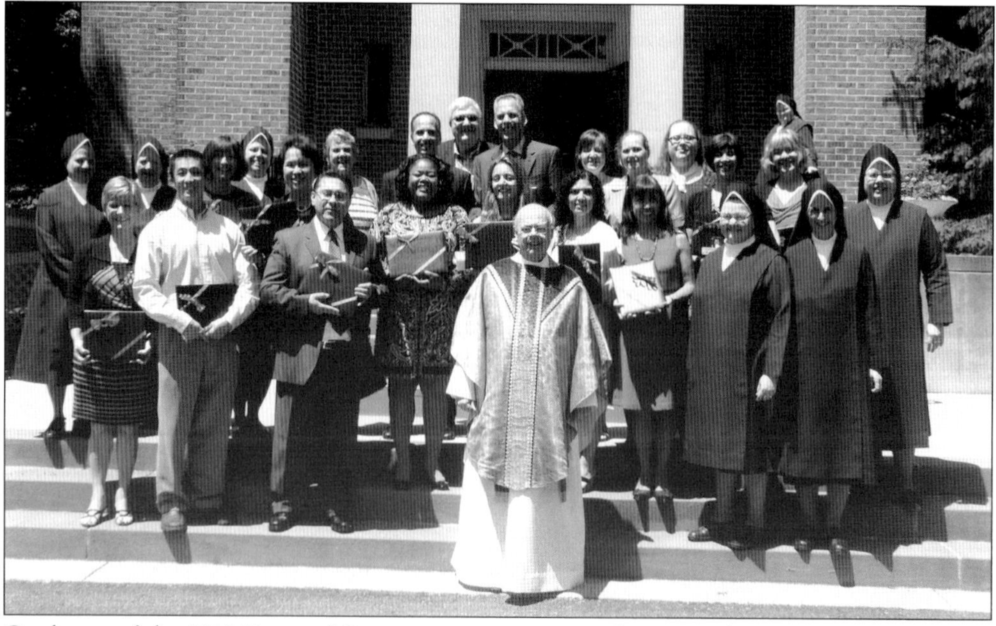

Graduates of the 2013 Roots of Caring program pose on the steps of St. Teresa's Chapel for a picture after receiving their certificates. This program is essential to train leaders in mission-based leadership for the future.

Five

Ninety Years of Caring for the Elderly

For 90 years now (September 3, 1929 to September 3, 2019), the Carmelite Sisters for the Aged and Infirm have been providing loving care to the elderly. From the first home for seven residents in the former rectory of St. Elizabeth's Parish in the Bronx, New York, to the 20 nursing homes, assisted living, and independent living facilities sponsored by and/or staffed by the Carmelite Sisters, Venerable Mother Angeline's vision of care has continued and expanded.

How proud she would be of her daughters in Carmel today as they have adapted over the years to the changing and challenging requirements of nursing care as they continue their mission of loving care for the elderly and the infirm. Today's residents are more acutely ill and require more specialized care than the first seven residents, who took on roles as gardener, cook, housekeeper, and others so that the sisters were free to go begging for money to keep them all fed and housed.

In response to a strategic planning process, which identified the need for facility support in an ever-changing health-care environment, the Carmelite System became a reality in 1999. It began as a service model and later passive parent, having the authority to influence operational and strategic changes to improve operating performance and implement programs to manage and operate under the new environment of health-care reform for member facilities. The system provides the following programs and services: Mission Enhancement, Resident Care and Clinical Program Support, Business Development, Collaboration and Networking Activities, Centralized Insurance Program, Finance and Operations Support, Human Resources, Contracting and Purchasing, Public Policy and Advocacy, Nurse Recruiting, Capital Project and Finance Support, Employee Benefits, Clinical Informatics, Grants Assistance, and Information Technology. Member facilities are sponsored by the Carmelite Sisters. The system also welcomes affiliates sponsored by other Catholic entities.

Now, in addition to providing nursing care for their residents, the sisters and their staff fundraise and write grant applications to help continue their ministry in the ever increasingly complicated world of medical costs and reimbursements. In all, the sisters today serve more than 4,000 residents.

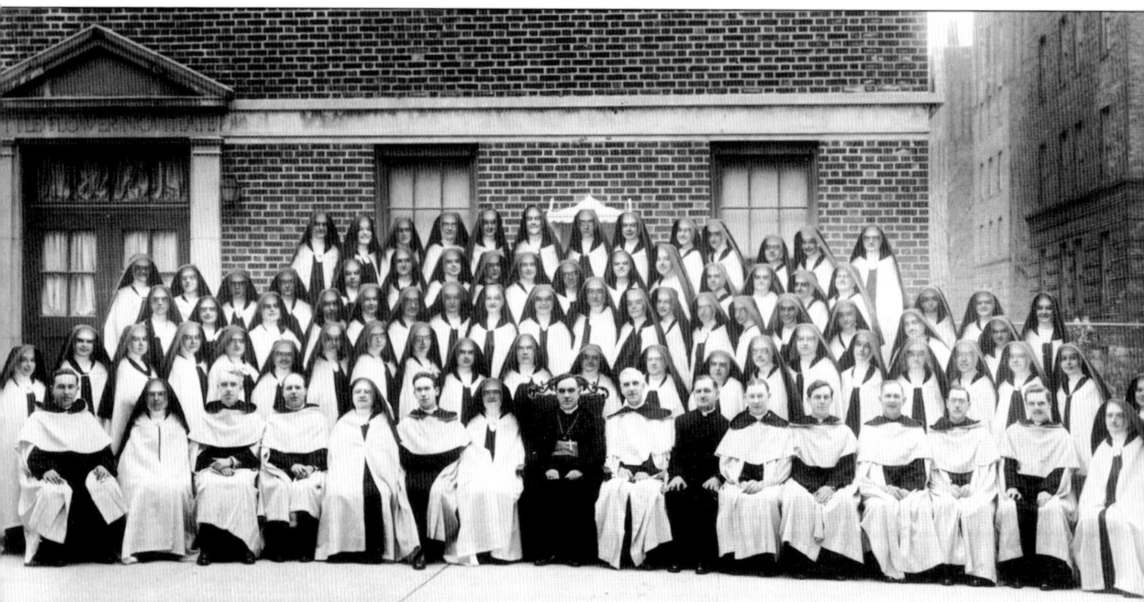

This is a photograph of professed sisters at St. Patrick's Home in the Bronx in 1940. The bishop in black in the middle of the first row is Bishop John Collins of Liberia, who was a guest at St. Patrick's at the time. Ten Carmelite priests also sit in the front row and were frequent guests, providing days of recollection for the sisters and helping to entertain the residents.

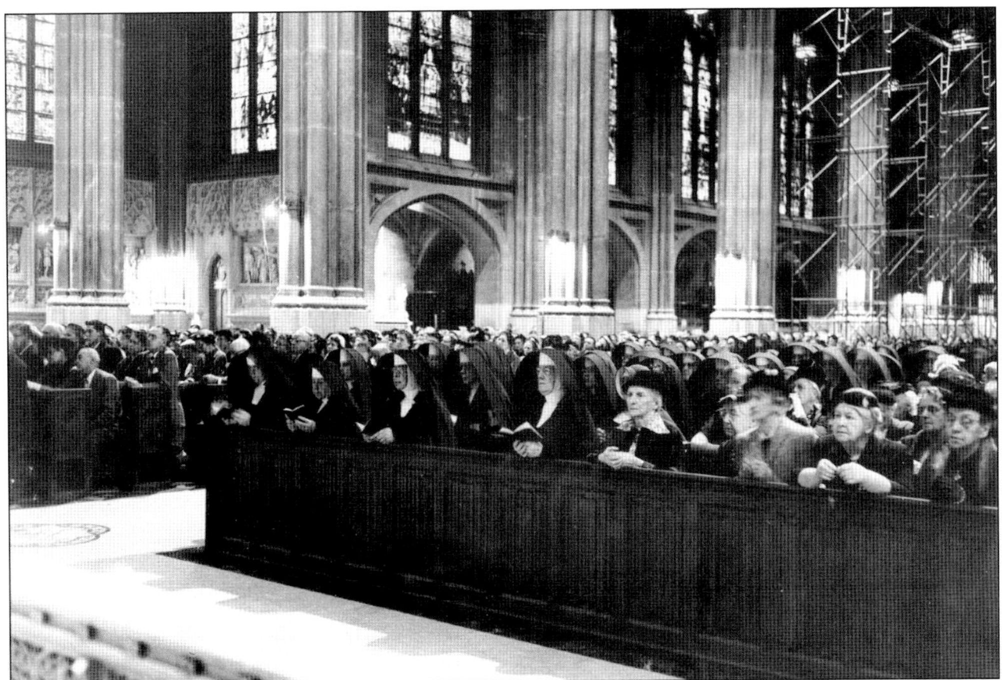

The Carmelite Sisters celebrated the 25th anniversary of their founding with a Mass at St. Patrick's Cathedral in New York City. Many of the residents of their various homes attended in support of the sisters on their silver anniversary.

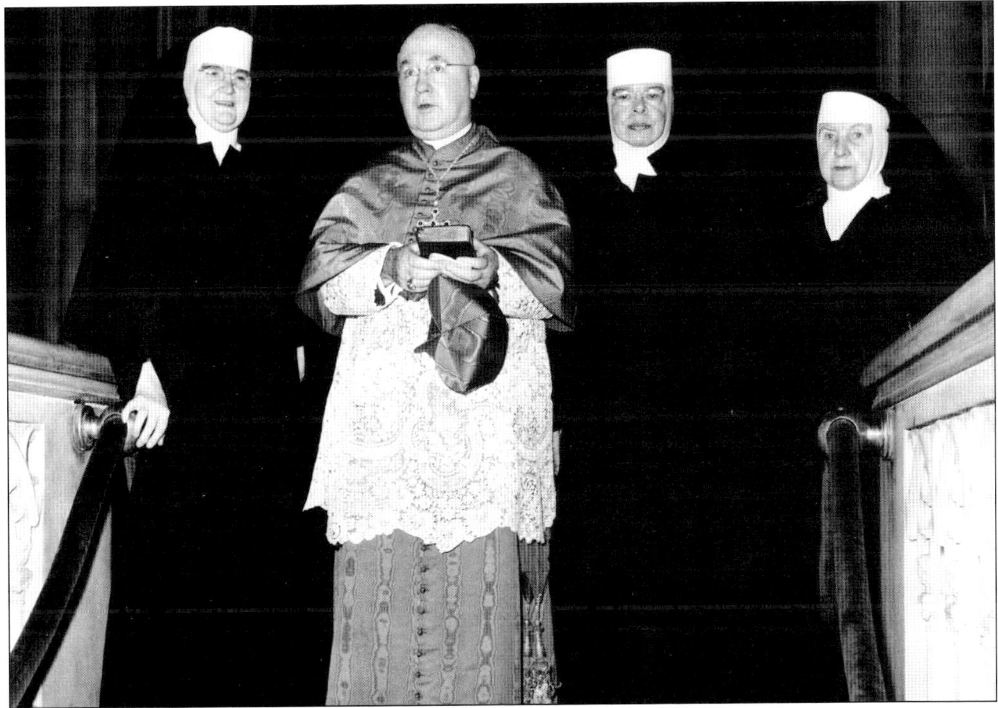

At the end of Mass, Mother Angeline (far left) posed for a picture with Cardinal Spellman, Mother Teresa, and Mother Colette, two of the original six sisters who were her early companions.

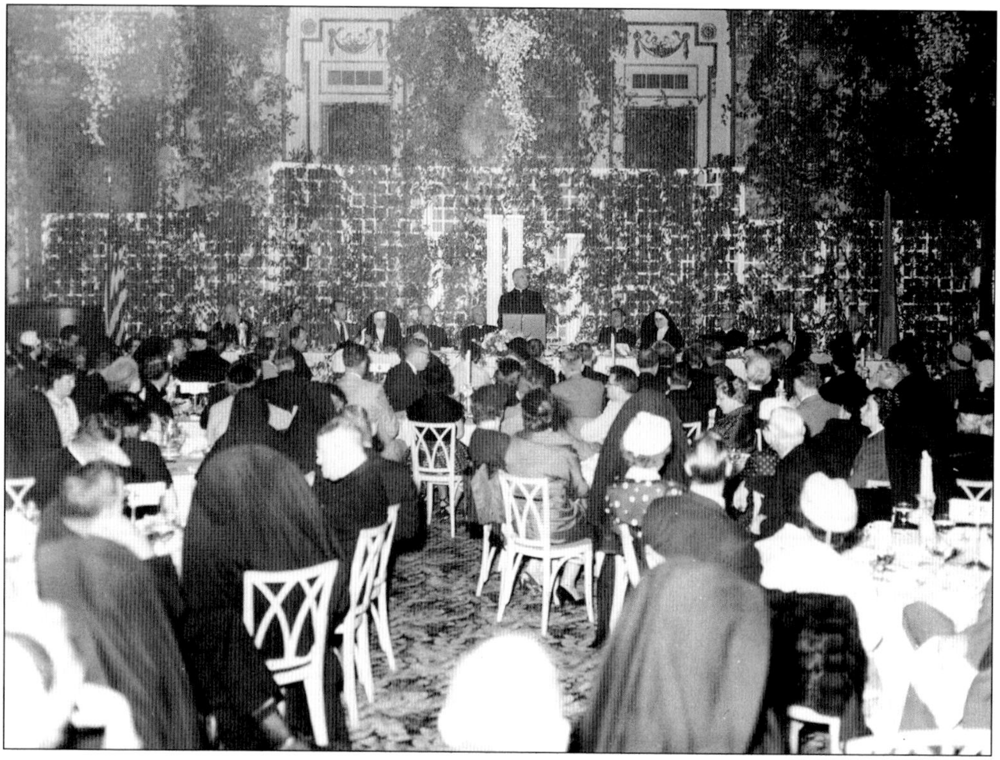

This is the ballroom of the Waldorf Astoria Hotel in New York City, where the 25th anniversary reception was held.

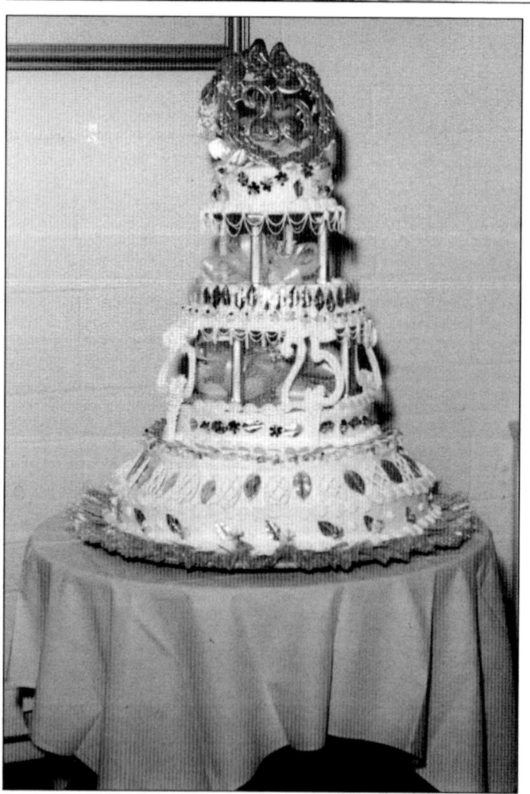

This is the 25th anniversary tiered cake that was served to reception attendees to mark the occasion.

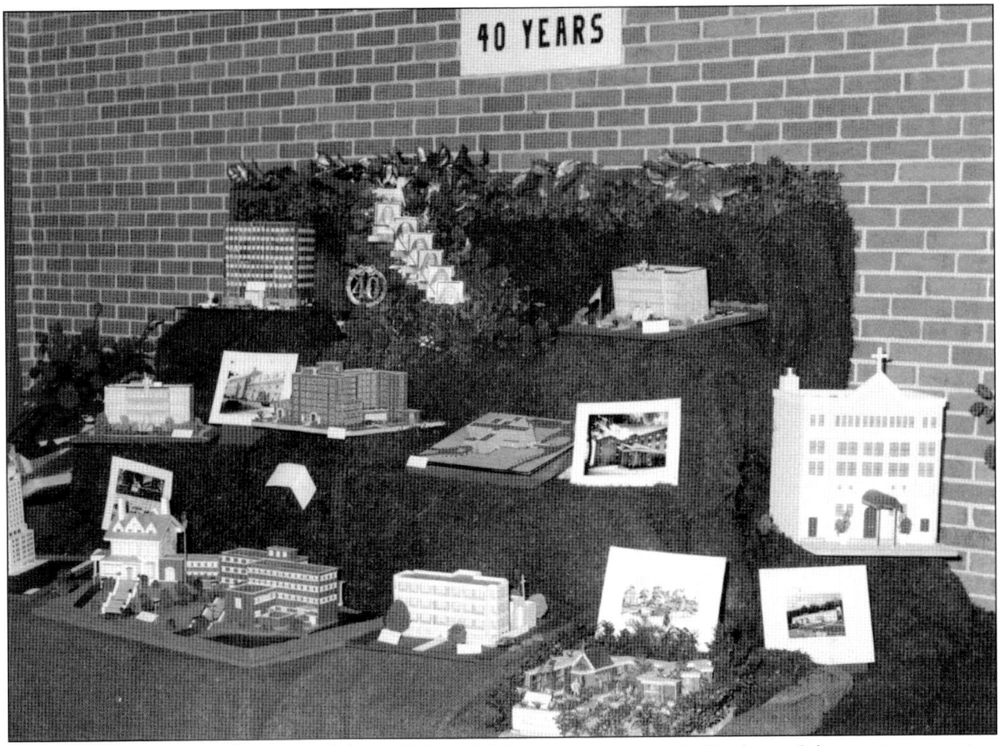

In 1969, the Carmelite Sisters celebrated their 40th anniversary with displays of the various nursing homes where they ministered. The display, entitled "40 Years of Progress," was made by the sisters and was set up in Carmel Hall, the all-purpose building located on the motherhouse grounds.

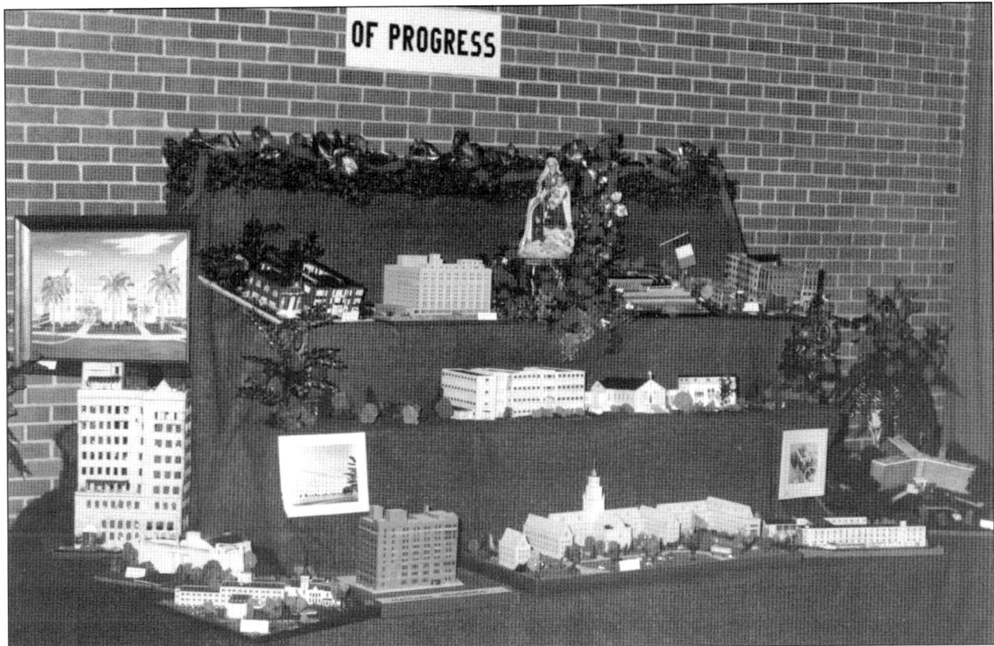

This is the second half of the display, showing the other homes sponsored or staffed by the Carmelite Sisters.

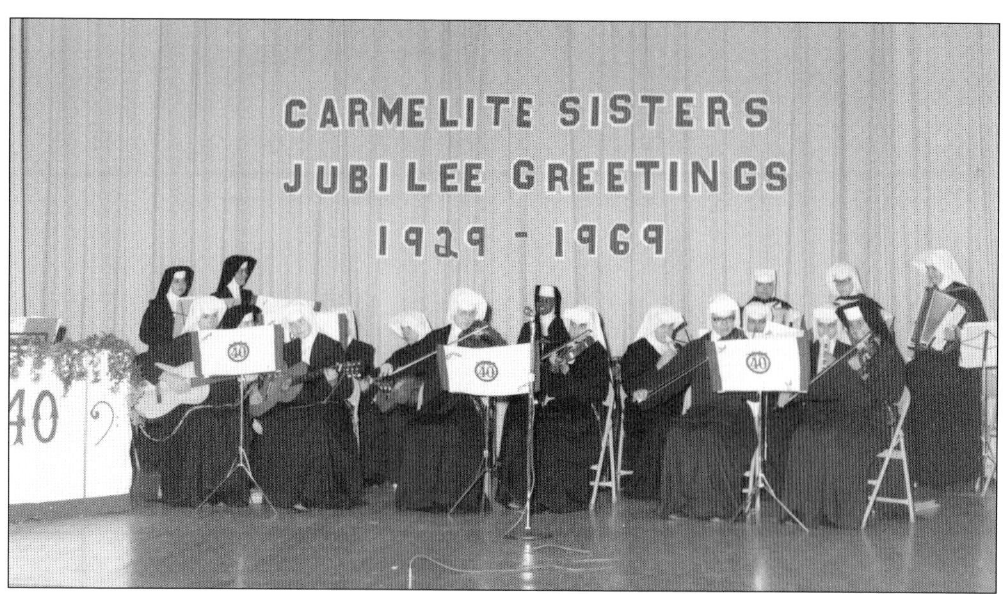

The Carmelite Orchestra gathered to entertain guests at the 40th anniversary reception.

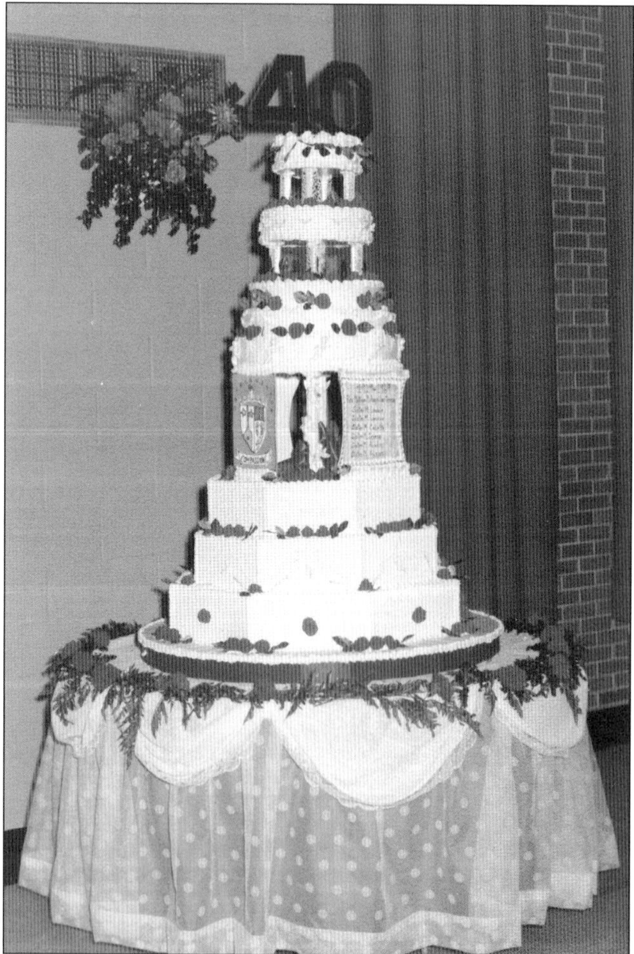

This is the tiered cake that was created for the 40th anniversary reception.

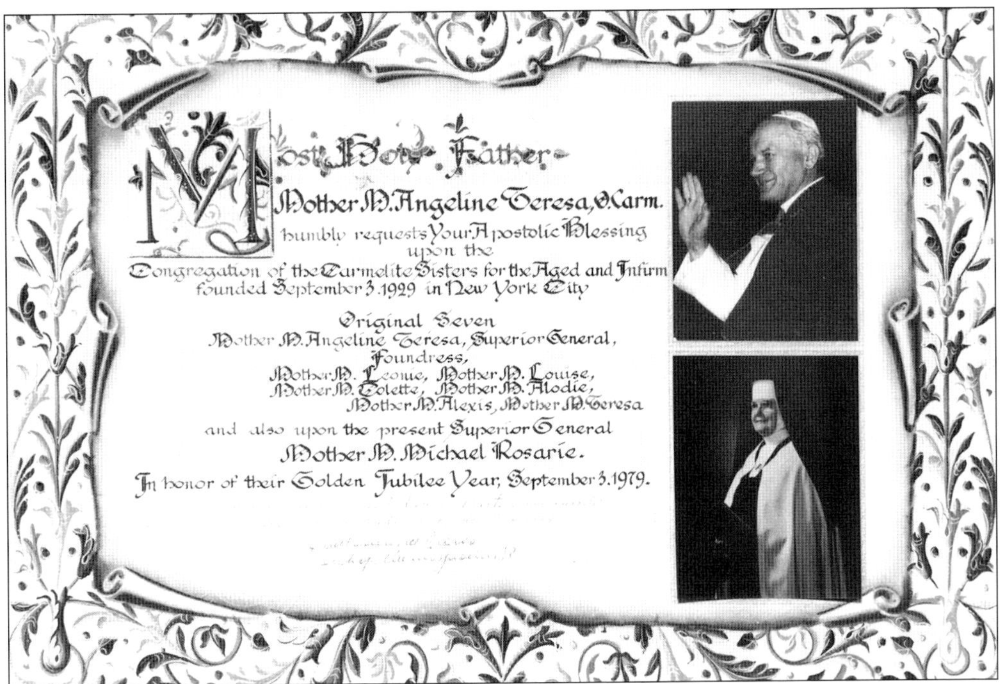
Most Holy Father
Mother M. Angeline Teresa, O.Carm.
humbly requests Your Apostolic Blessing
upon the
Congregation of the Carmelite Sisters for the Aged and Infirm
founded September 3. 1929 in New York City
Original Seven
Mother M. Angeline Teresa, Superior General,
Foundress,
Mother M. Leonie, Mother M. Louise,
Mother M. Colette, Mother M. Alodie,
Mother M. Alexis, Mother M. Teresa
and also upon the present Superior General
Mother M. Michael Rosarie.
In honor of their Golden Jubilee Year, September 3. 1979.

For the 50th anniversary in 1979, Mother Angeline requested a papal blessing on the original seven sisters and on Mother M. Michael Rosarie, who had been elected as Mother Angeline's successor in 1978 after Mother Angeline stepped down due to illness.

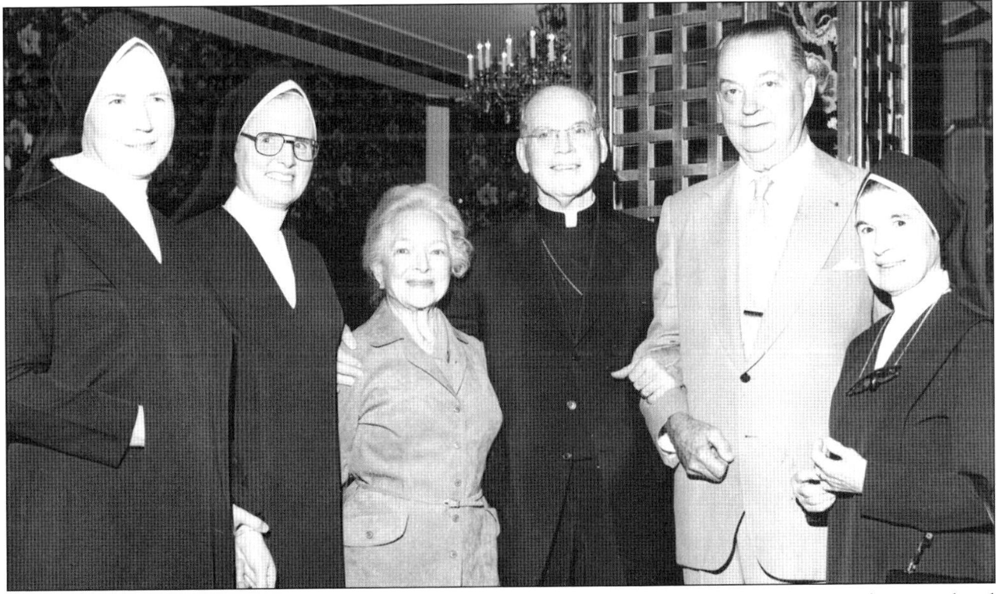

Present at the reception were, from left to right, Mother Kathleen Rosarie; Mother Michael Rosarie the actress Helen Hayes, who was a great supporter of the sisters; Terence Cardinal Cooke; Dr. Howard Rusk, who founded the Rusk Rehabilitation Institute and worked closely with the sisters to develop physical therapy and occupational therapy programs in their nursing homes; and Mother Bernadette de Lourdes, author of the book *Where Somebody Cares*, which served as a guide for the management of nursing homes in the United States.

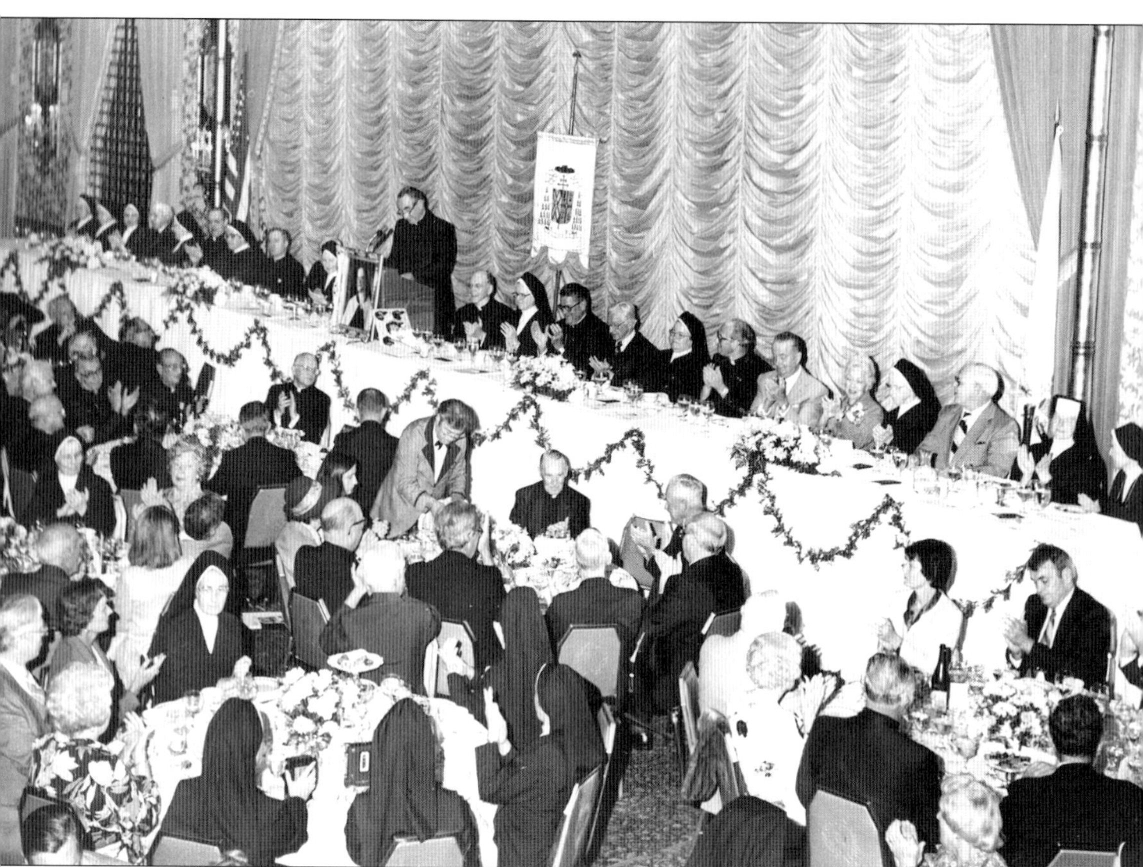

This is an overhead view of the guests and the dais during the 50th anniversary reception, also held at the Waldorf Astoria Hotel.

This is the save-the-date announcement for the 75th anniversary Mass and reception afterwards at the Pierre Hotel.

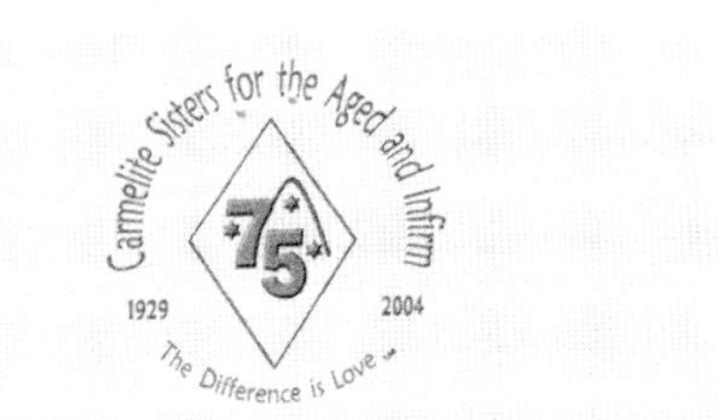

Join the Carmelite Sisters for the Aged and Infirm
as we joyfully celebrate
75 Years
in service to God and the Church

Saturday, October 23, 2004
Mass at 10 A.M.
Cathedral of Saint Patrick
50th Street & 5th Ave.
New York City

Luncheon immediately following at
The Pierre
Fifth Avenue and 61st Street
New York City

Formal invitation to follow
For journal information contact co-chairs:
Sr. M. Kevin Patricia or Sr. M. Anthony de Lourdes
518-537-5000

St. Patrick's Cathedral was filled to capacity as the procession of priests worked its way down the main aisle.

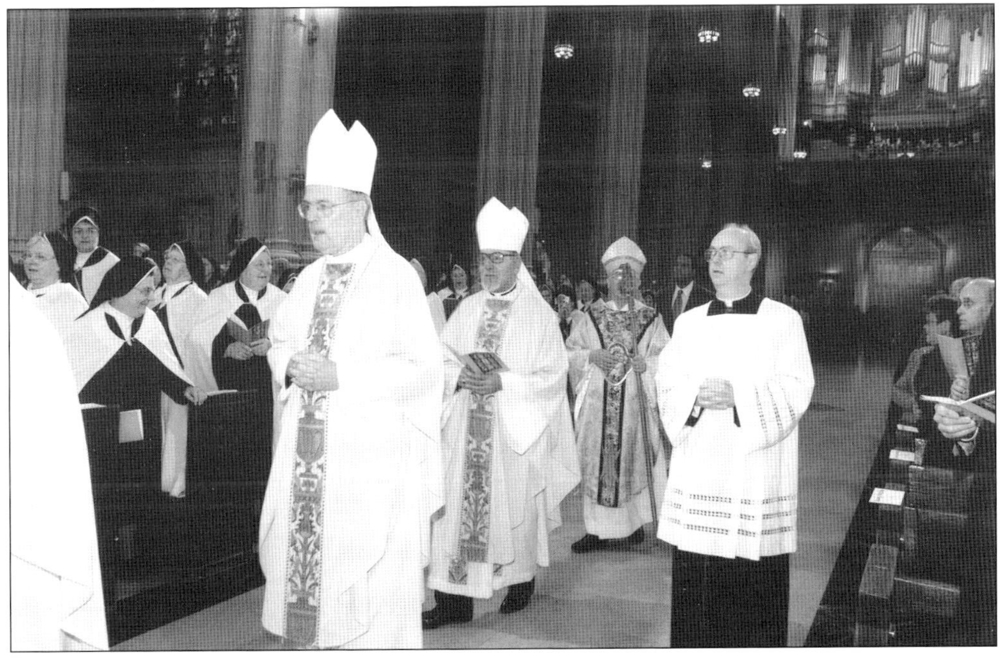

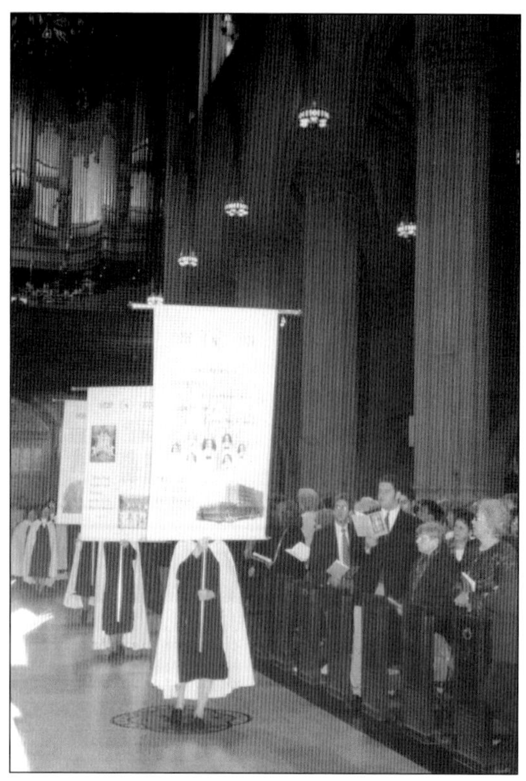

The sisters processed in, carrying three banners. The first represented Mother Angeline and her six companions above the first foundation, St. Patrick's Home; the second banner portrayed Avila, the beloved motherhouse and grounds of the Carmelite Sisters; and the third portrayed a sculpture of the elderly with Jesus and a quote from Mother Angeline, who always told the sisters, "Try to be kinder than kindness itself."

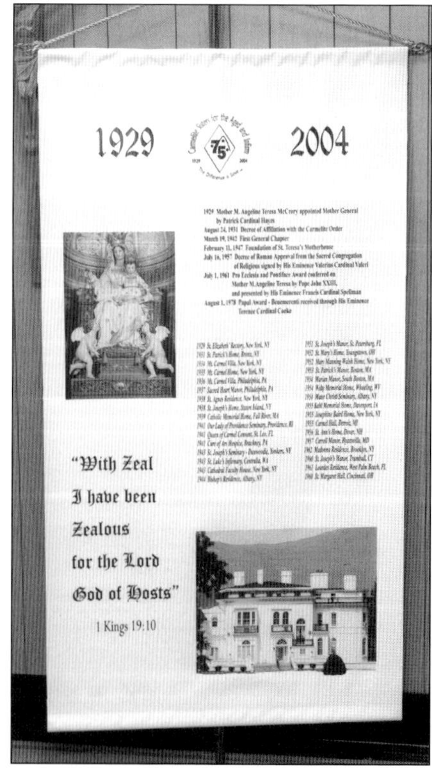

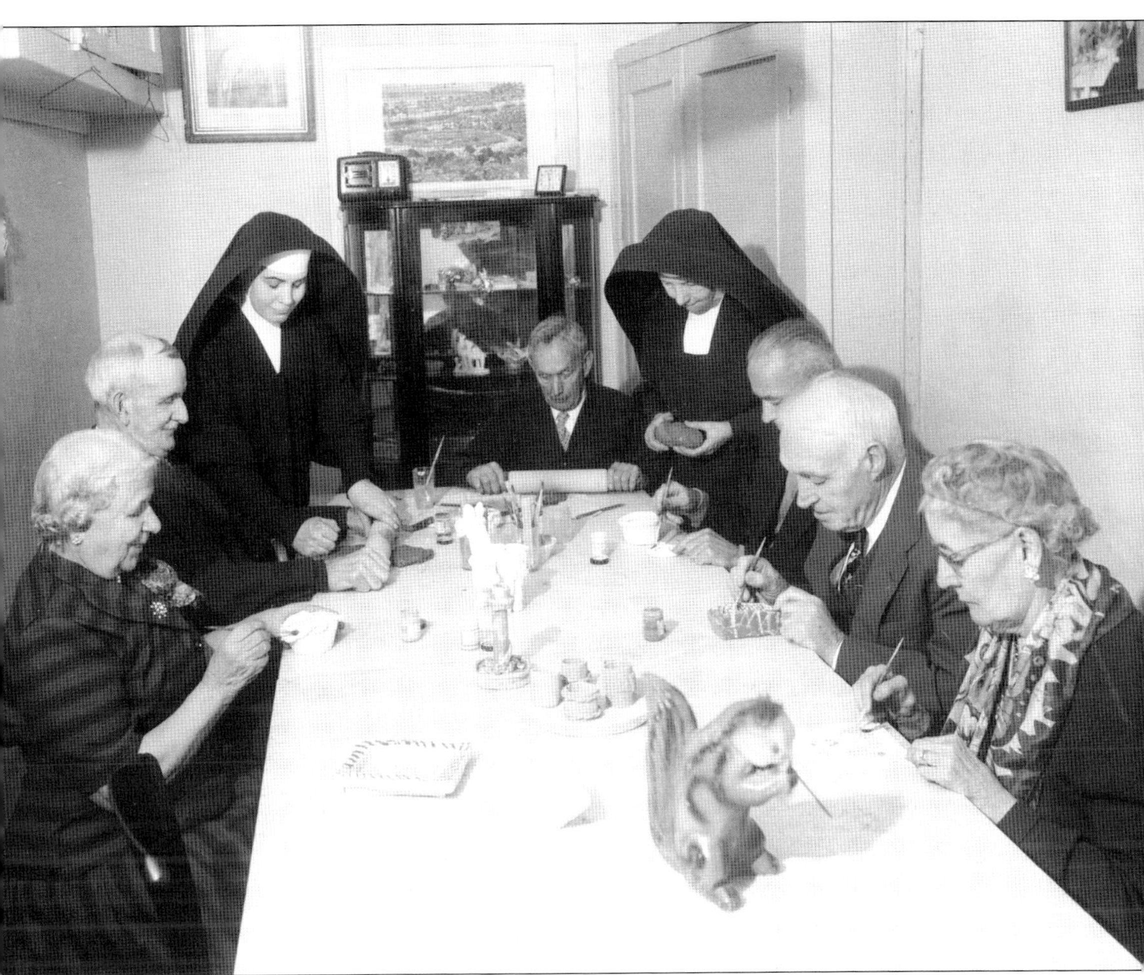

The sisters are seen here in the early days working with the residents at St. Patrick's Home on their activities.

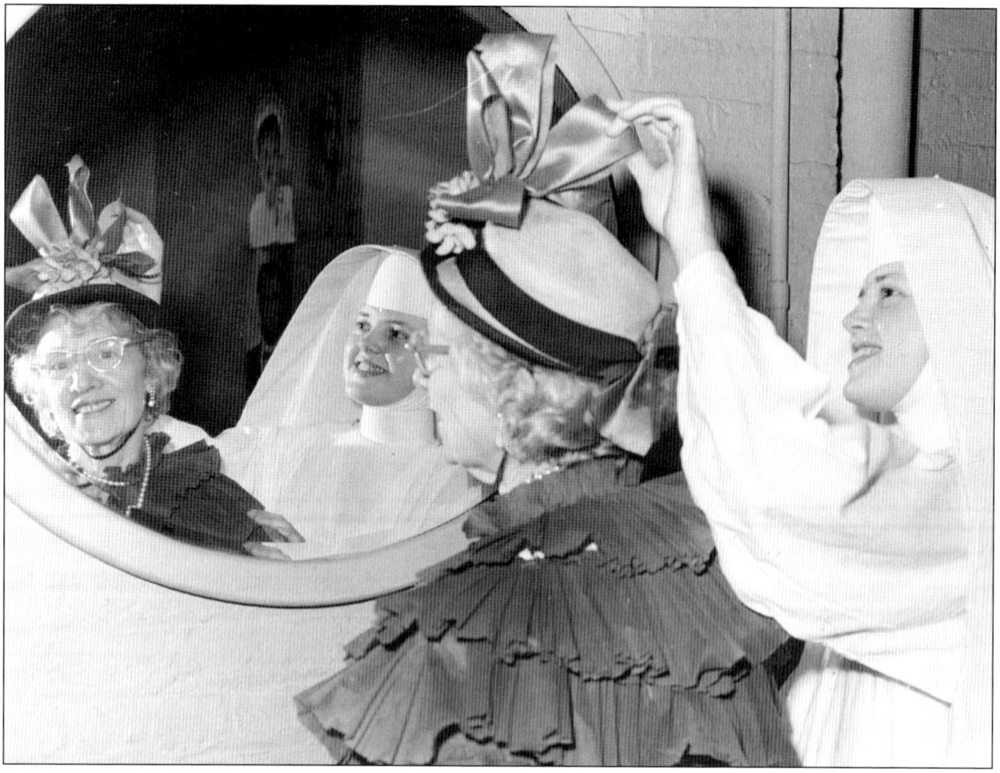

A resident has her hat adjusted by Sr. Patricia Ann of the Assumption before she goes out for a special event.

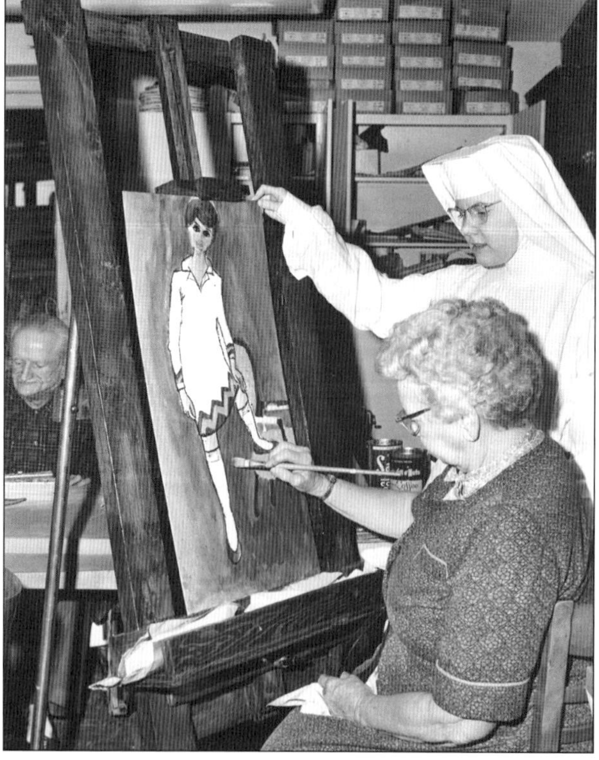

Sr. Celine Marian admires the work of a resident in the art room.

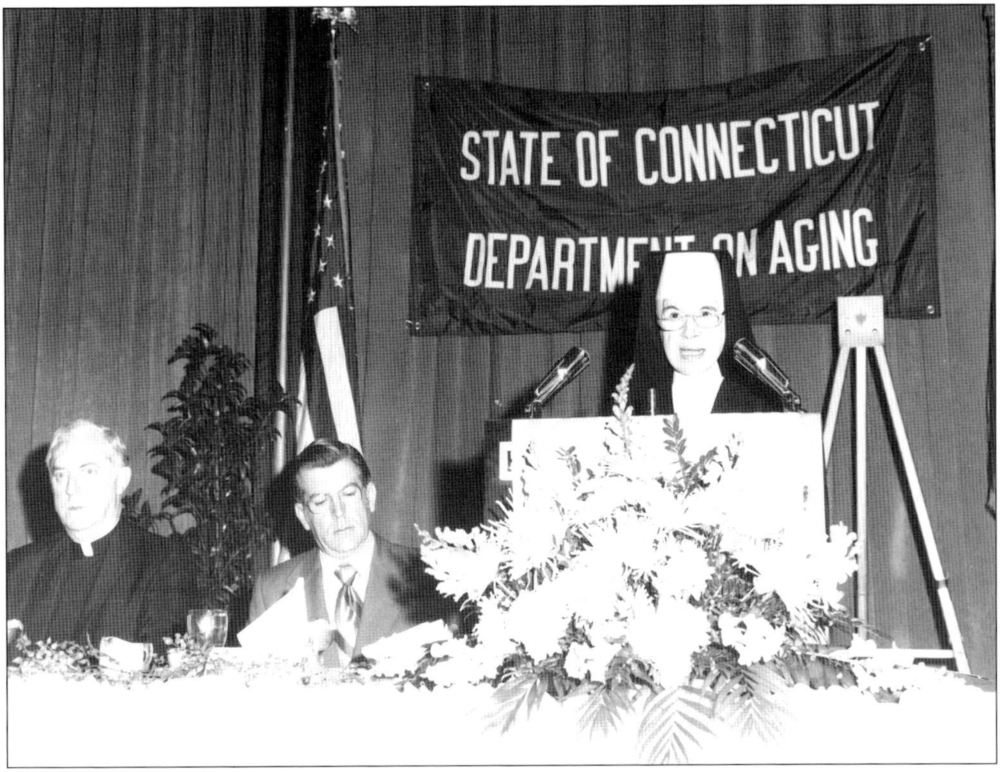

Mother Bernadette de Lourdes, who was the administrator of St. Joseph's Manor nursing home in Trumbull, Connecticut, was appointed by Gov. Thomas Meskill to be the very first commissioner on the aging in the state of Connecticut. She served in that capacity from 1960 to 1975.

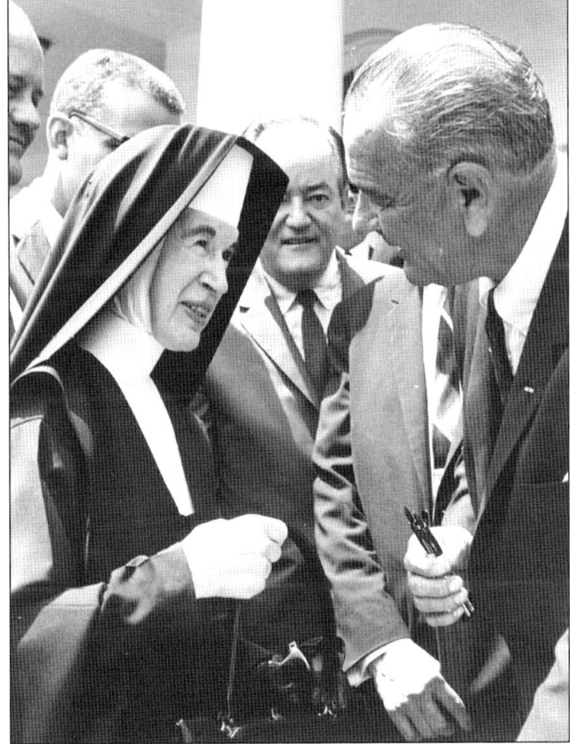

Mother Bernadette is seen here with Pres. Lyndon B. Johnson when he signed House Bill 3708 authorizing the development of programs for the elderly and the Administration on Aging.

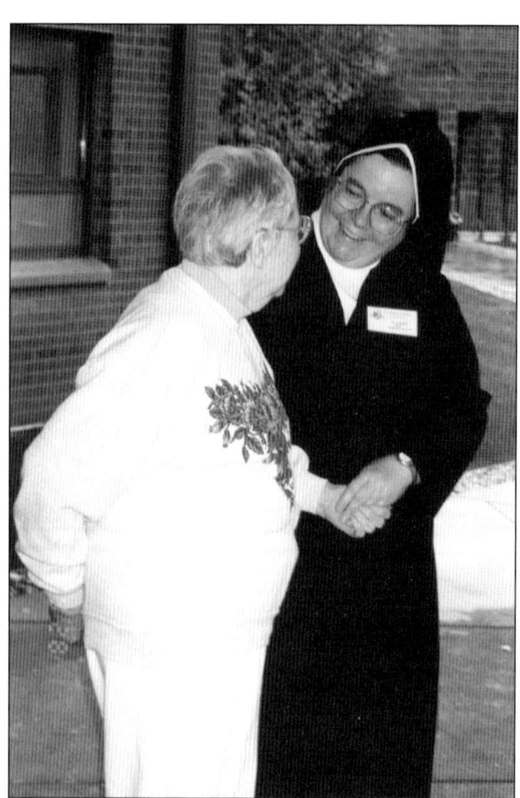

Sr. Jeanne Francis takes a resident for a walk outside St. Patrick's Residence in Naperville, Illinois.

Sr. Colette of the Assumption spends some quality time with a resident. Sr. Colette, from Ireland, was the niece of Mother Colette, one of the sisters who left the Little Sisters of the Poor along with Mother Angeline.

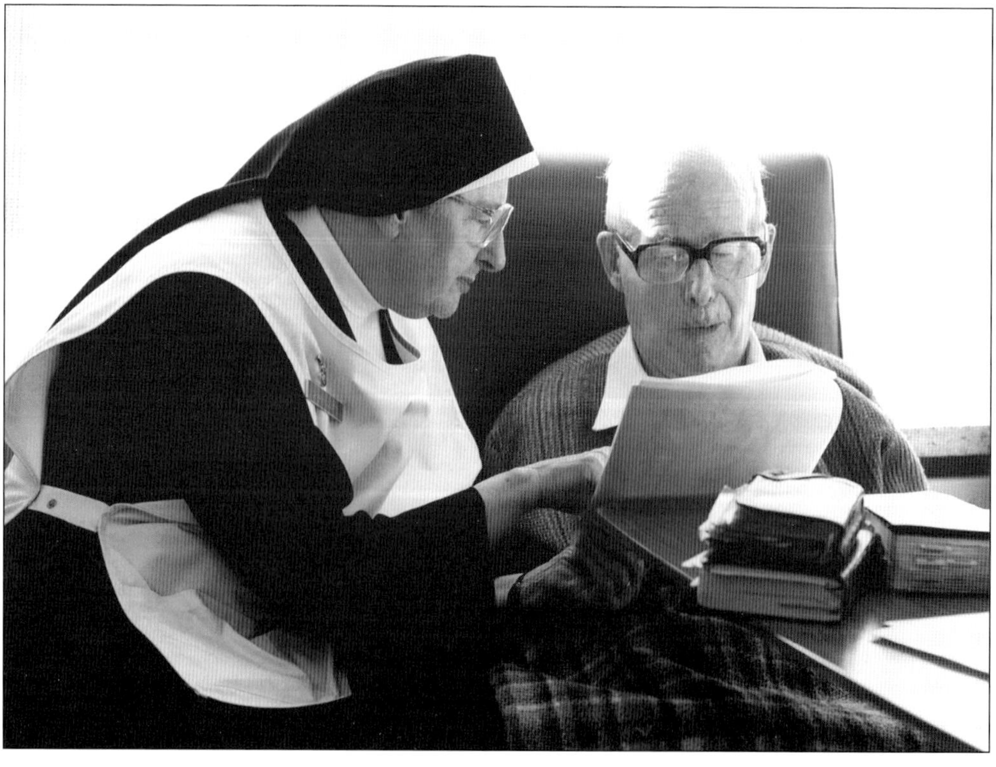

At center, Sr. Patrick Michael, buoyant in spirit, dances with a resident at an outdoor party as Sr. Marcella Bean looks on.

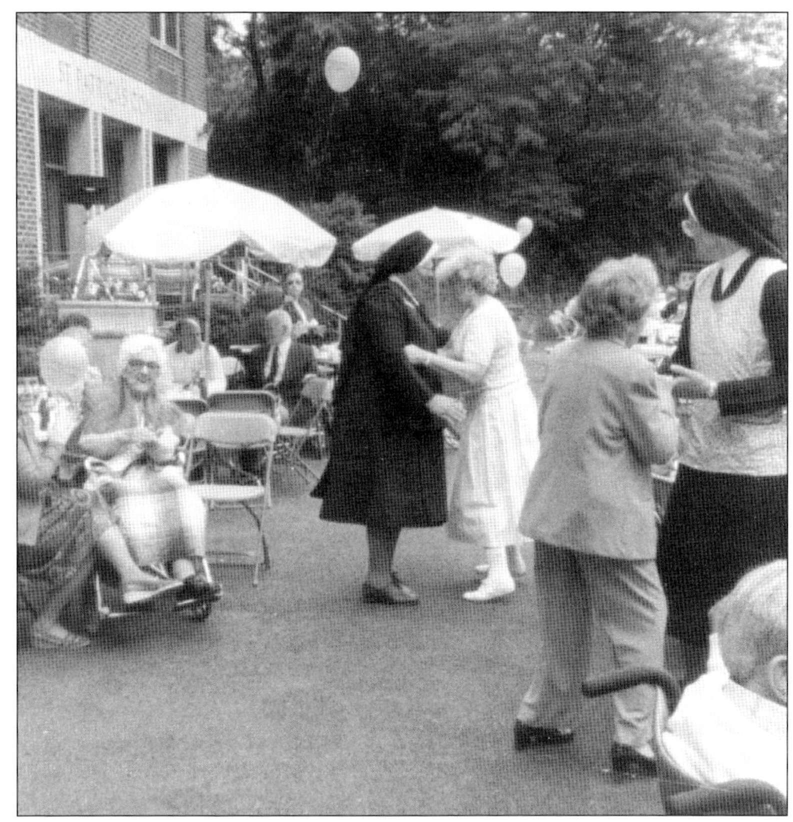

Sr. Patricia Francis and an employee at Our Lady's Manor fold towels and sheets in the laundry. She was known for all the dolls that she would knit for the facilities to sell in their gift shops or at fundraising events.

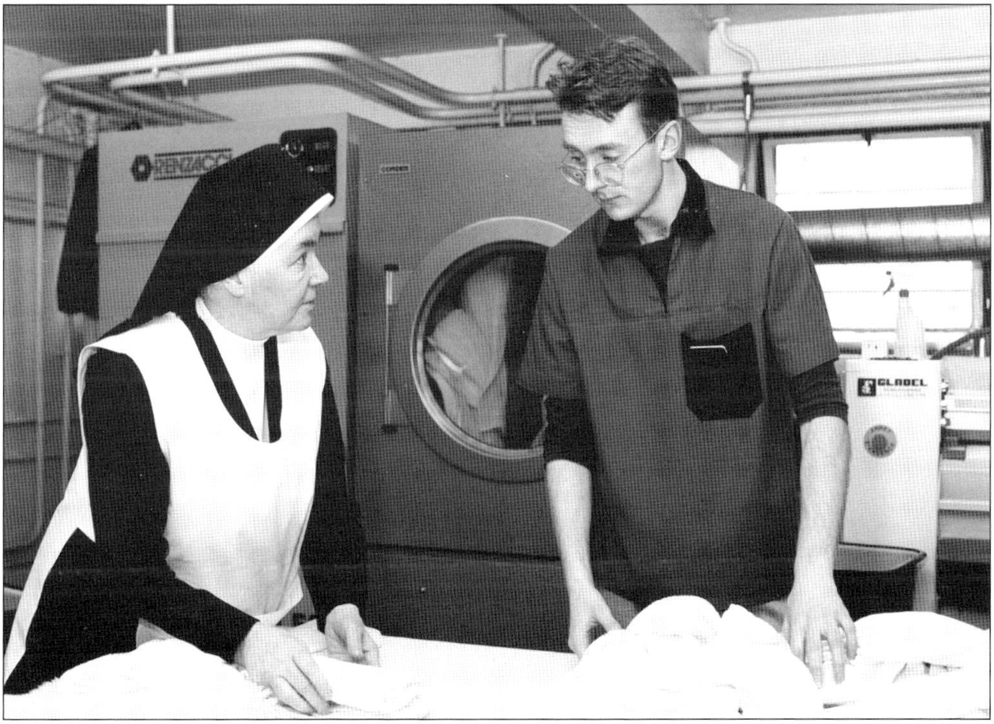

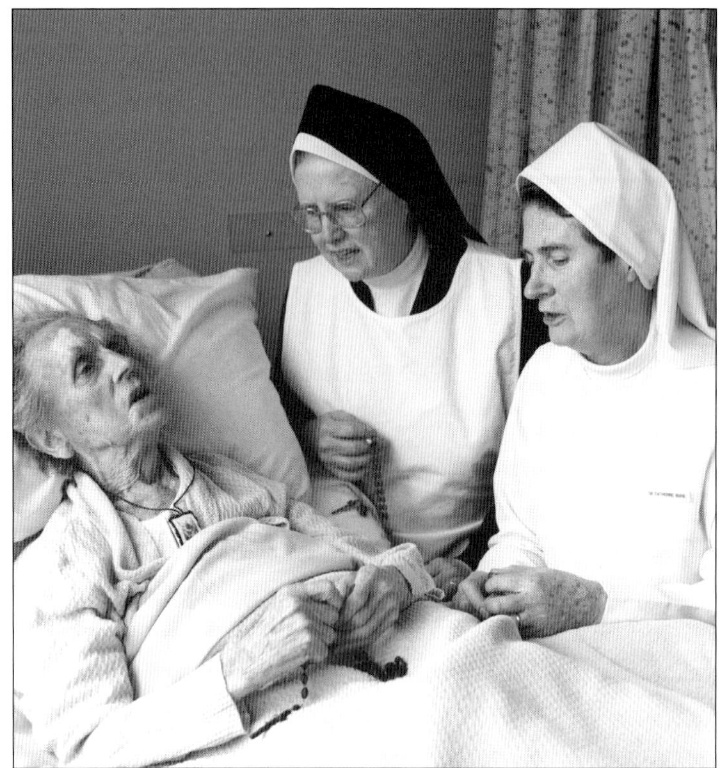

The Carmelite Sisters have a custom of praying at the bedside of a dying resident. They wish to provide love and support to residents and families in this last journey. In this photograph, Mother Michael Rosarie and Sr. Catherine Marie pray the rosary with a resident at Our Lady's Manor in Dalkey, Ireland.

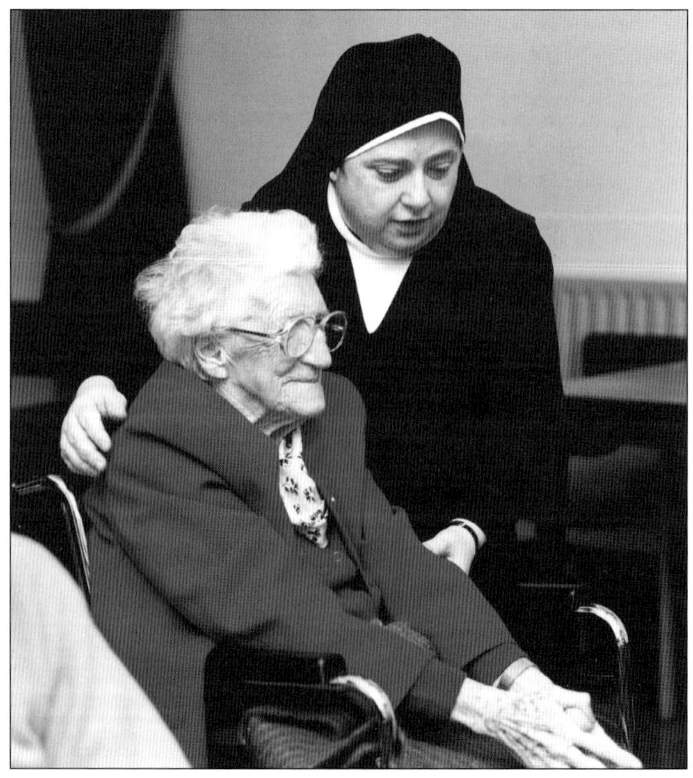

Sr. Deirdre Ferguson helps a resident do her exercises.

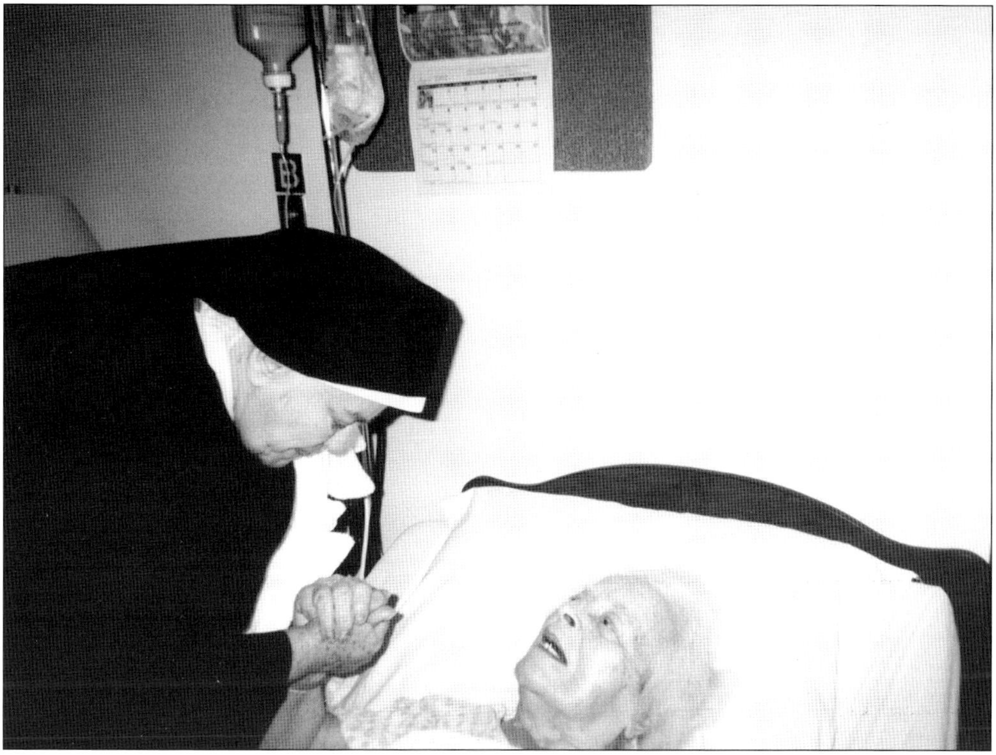

Sr. Mary Joseph prays with a resident at her bedside. Sr. Mary Joseph completed the Geriatric Spiritual Care Certificate program, and provided pastoral care services to the residents in her various missions.

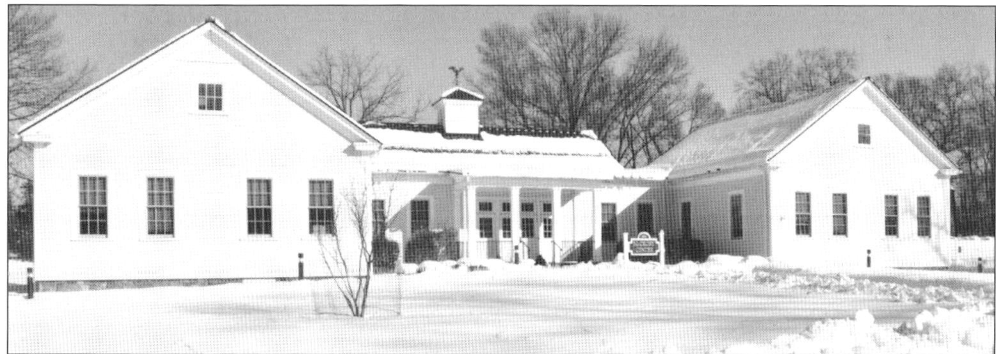

Pictured here is the McCrory Center, which houses the Carmelite System on the motherhouse grounds. The system, which celebrates its 20th anniversary in 2019, provides support to the facilities to help the sisters face the ever-changing health-care environment.

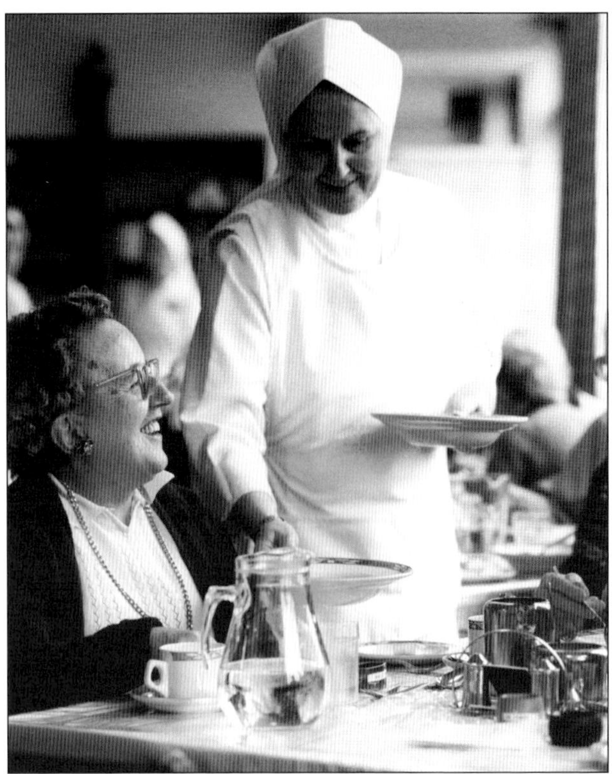

Sr. Mary Therese of Jesus shares a laugh with resident Deirdre Fitzpatick as she serves her some soup at Our Lady's Manor in Dalkey, Ireland.

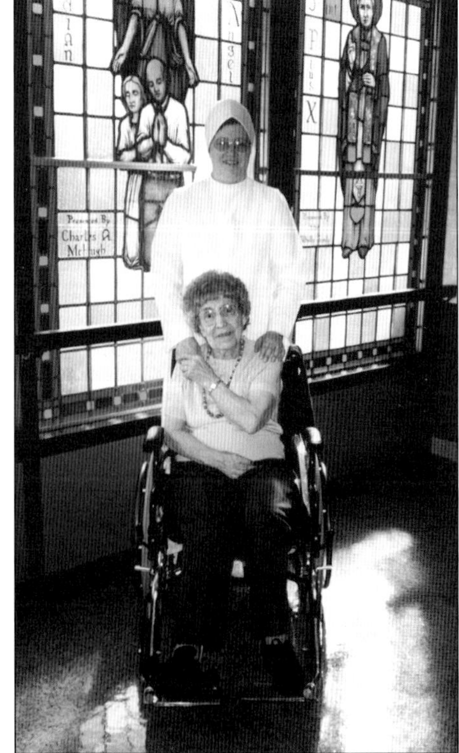

Sr. Theresa Pfeffer is pictured here with a resident in the chapel of Sacred Heart Manor, where she was stationed before becoming assistant director of clinical services at the Carmelite System.

The sisters know how to have a good time as well. Sr. Ambrose of the Holy Angels is seen dressed as a leprechaun alongside Sr. Elias of Mount Carmel, also decked out in green, as they celebrate St. Patrick's Day.

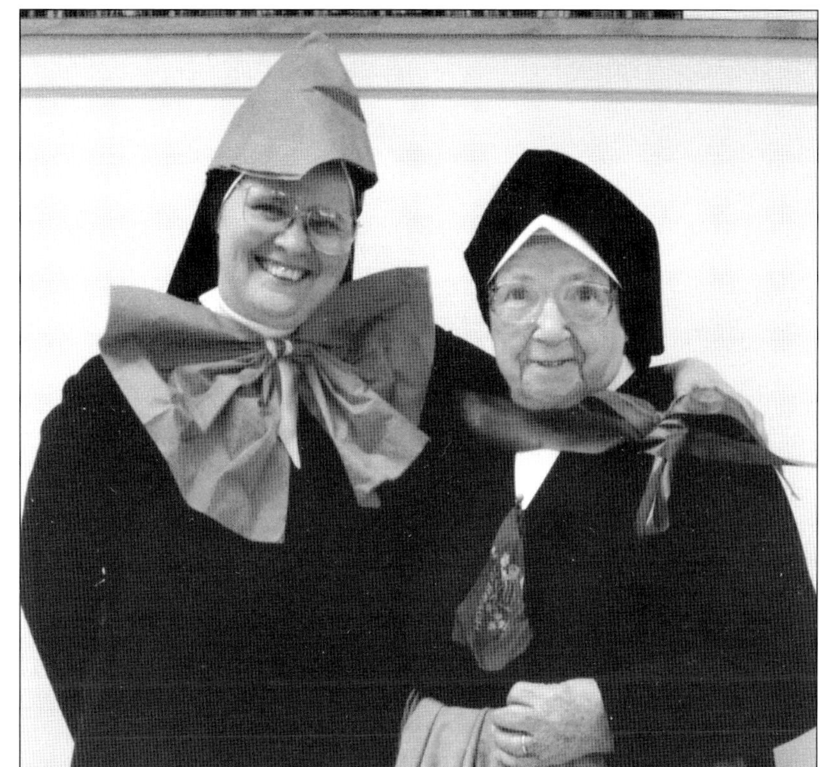

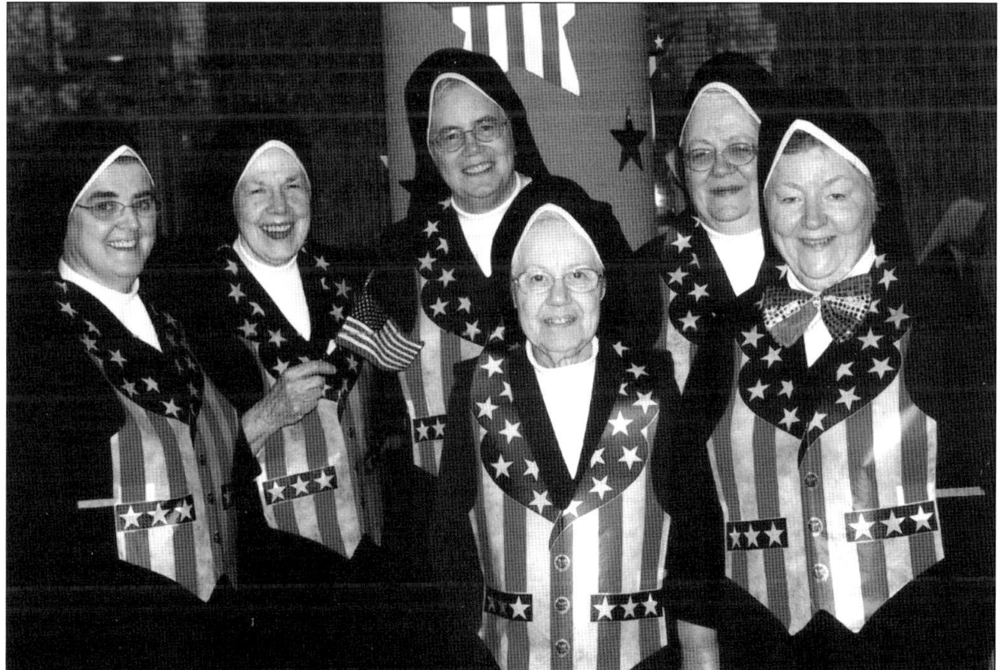

The Fourth of July is an occasion for celebration as well. From left to right are Sr. Kathleen John Immaculate, Sr. Barbara Higgins, Sr. Maureen Carroll, Sr. Joseph Angela (foreground), Sr. Winifred Angeline, and Sr. Kevin Patricia of the Holy Angels.

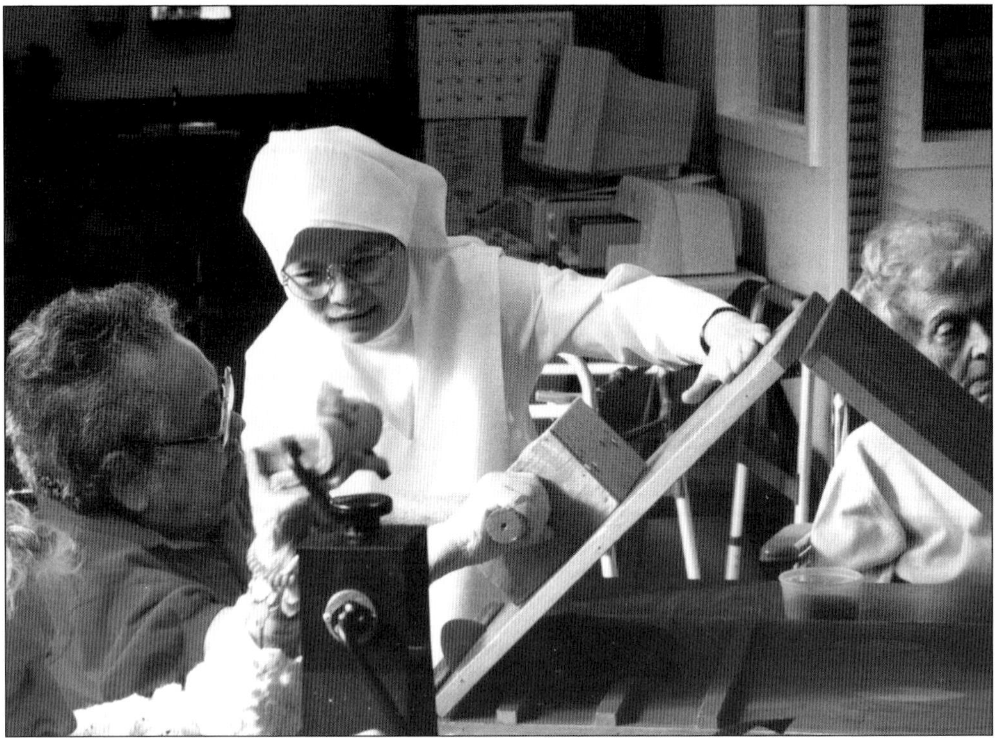

Sr. Theresa of the Eucharist helps residents with their projects.

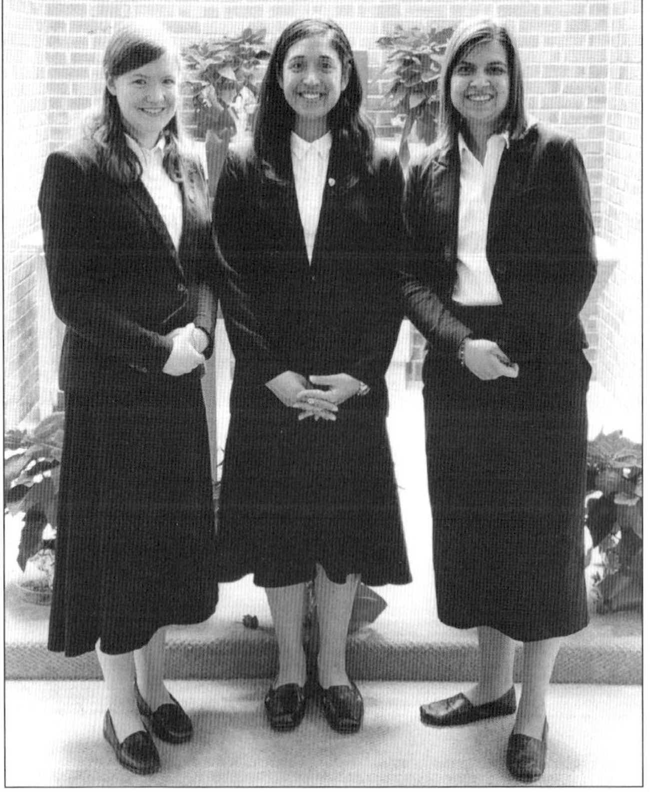

The vitality of the congregation can be seen in the smiles of the postulants who entered the community in September 2018. The enthusiasm of Sr. Sharon Mullin, Sr. Doris Benitez, and Sr. Morgan Mondello can be felt by all as they begin their journey in Carmel.

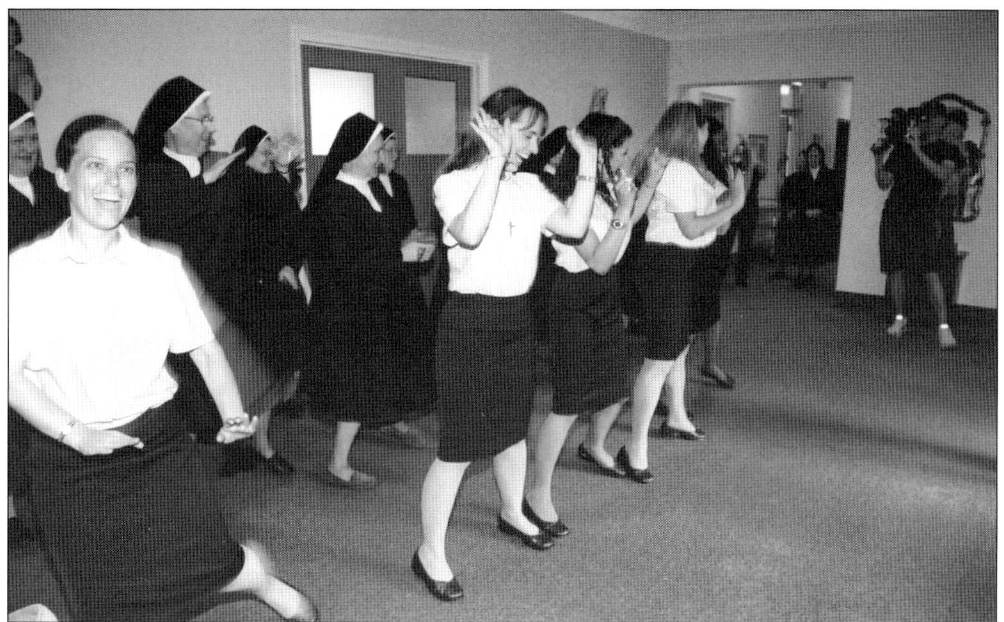

In November 2014, the Lifetime network debuted an all-new series titled *The Sisterhood: Becoming Nuns*. The series follows five young women during the initial discernment phase of entering religious life as Catholic sisters. One of the convents visited during the series is that of the Carmelite Sisters for the Aged and Infirm. The sisters were able to interact with and offer guidance to these young women as they continued their journeys.

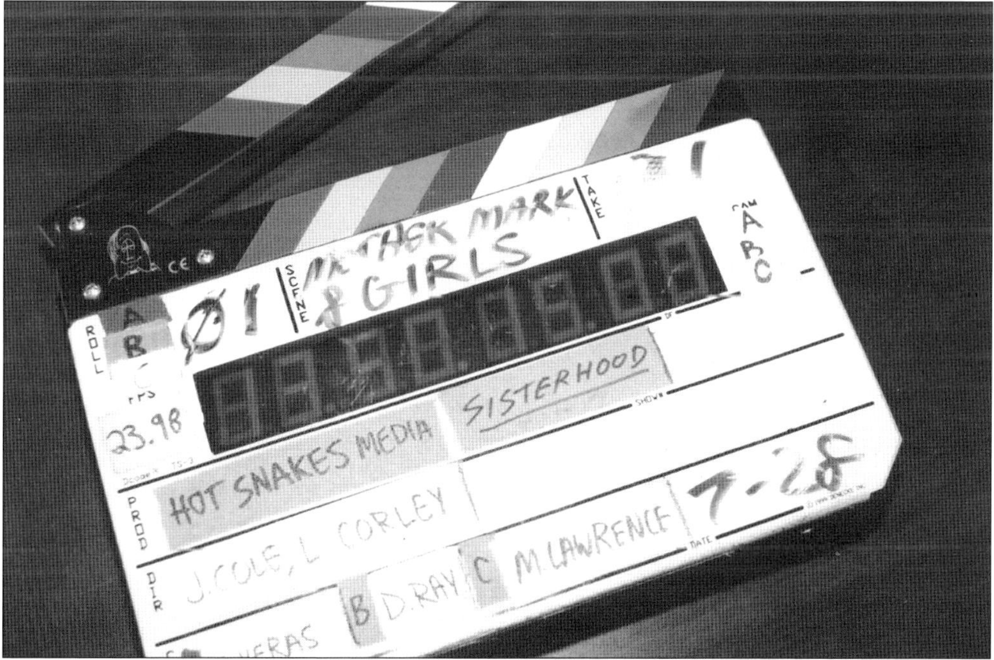

This is one of the clapperboards used during the production of *The Sisterhood*. It was for the scene with Mother Mark speaking with the young women.

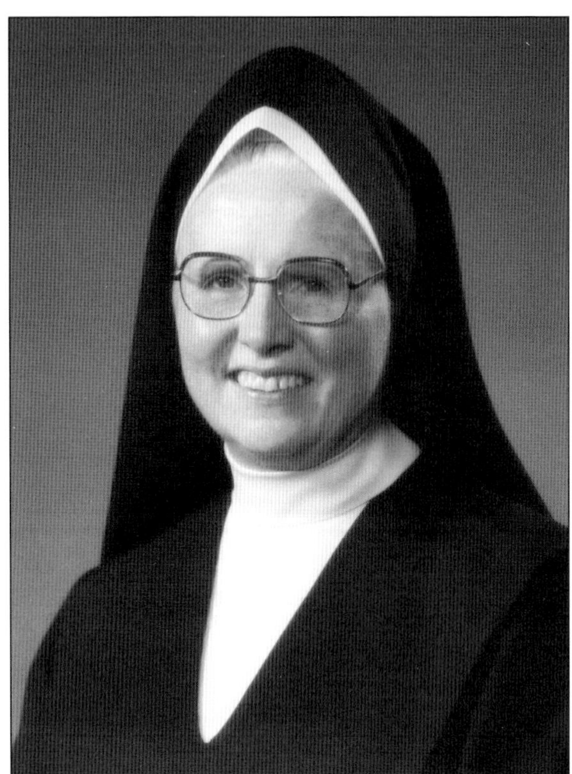

Mother Michael Rosarie served two terms as superior general from September 1978 to September 1990. She had been vicar general of the congregation since 1972. In 1978, she was elected to follow Mother Angeline, who was aging and declined to be considered again for the position. Mother Michael had ministered in lab and X-ray and administration before her election as vicar general.

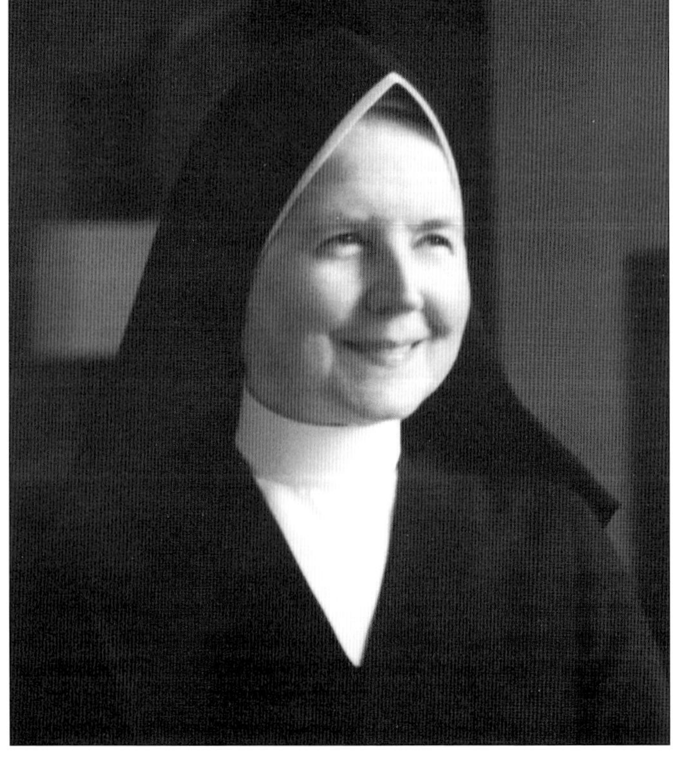

Mother Kathleen Rosarie served one term as superior general from September 1990 to 1996. Mother Kathleen had been administrator of two homes in Boston, where she acquired vast experience in updating and constructing facilities. She was elected to the general council in 1976 upon the death of Mother Brendan and was vicar general before her election as superior general.

Mother Suzanne served two terms as superior general from 1996 to 2008. Mother Suzanne had been postulant director, secretary general, and member of the general council before her election as superior general. She now coordinates pastoral care services at Carmel Richmond Nursing Home on Staten Island, New York.

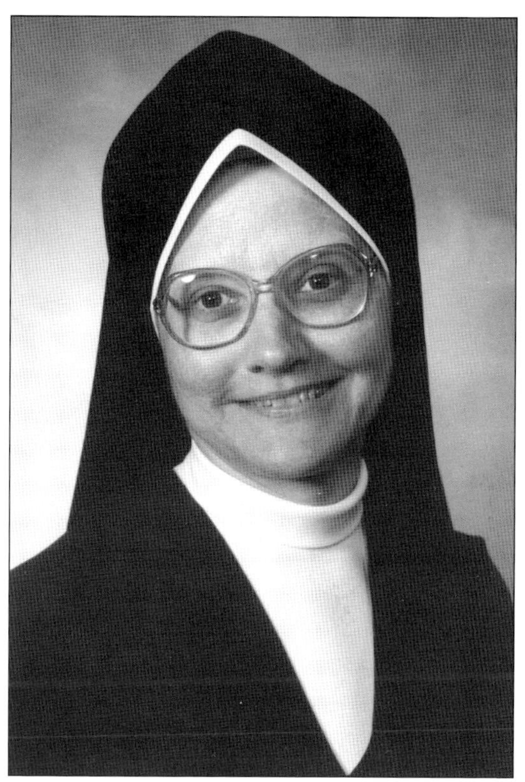

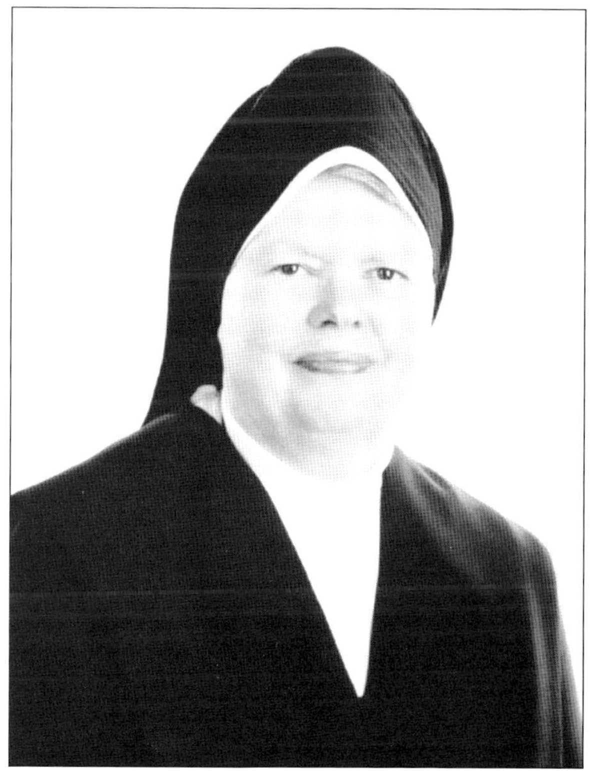

Mother Mark Louis Anne is the current prioress general and is serving in her second term, which will end in September 2020. Mother Mark had previously been a social worker, administrator, and member of the general council before being elected to her current position.

List of Carmelite Sisters for the Aged and Infirm

Sr. Alice Webster
Sr. Angelica Rose Marie Mora
Sr. Ann Dailey
Sr. Ann Elizabeth Brown
Sr. Ann McCartney
Sr. Anne Patricia Ruiz
Sr. Barbara Francis Higgins
Sr. Barbara Maloy
Sr. Bernadette Marie O'Sullivan
Sr. Bernadette Mary Lee
Sr. Bernadine Anna Skasko
Sr. Carol Nolan
Sr. Carolyn Therese Keane
Sr. Deirdre Mary Ferguson
Sr. Diane Marie Mack
Sr. Eileen Mary Fitzsimmons
Sr. Elena Castaneda
Sr. Helena of Mary Rocolcol
Sr. Jacinta Mary Hirner
Sr. Jean Ann Davis
Sr. Joan Mary Lewis
Sr. Joseph Angelina Marie Castano
Sr. Leda Veronica Domino
Sr. Lois Ann Wetzel
Sr. Luke Mary Angeline Lukose
Sr. M. Patricia Eileen Rosinski
Sr. M. Ambrose of the Holy Angels Niznik
Sr. M. Anthony de Lourdes Veilleux
Sr. M. Anthony Rosarie DiOrio
Sr. M. Bernadette Murphy
Sr. M. Bernadette Therese De Lourdes Reilly
Sr. M. Brendan Rosarie O'Brien
Sr. M. Brendan Sean Phillips
Sr. M. Brigid De Lourdes Riley
Sr. M. Carmel Cecilia O'Connor
Sr. M. Carmelita of Jesus Zawada
Sr. M. Catherine Angeline Hinkle
Sr. M. Catherine Leighton
Sr. M. Charlotte Michael Smolik
Sr. M. Christopher Jude Pineault
Sr. M. Clare of the Holy Angels Jagenow
Sr. M. Constance de Lourdes Richards
Sr. M. Cyril Methodius Kasper
Sr. M. Dolores Courtney
Sr. M. Edwin Thomas Debany
Sr. M. Elizabeth Ann Soderquist
Sr. M. Ellen Bernadette Magano
Sr. M. Eulaliae Angeline George
Sr. M. Fidelis Therese Fay
Sr. M. Francis Cecile Marcinak
Sr. M. Francis Clare of All Saints Magano
Sr. M. Francis of All Saints Meno
Sr. M. Francis Patrick Casey
Sr. M. Francis Pio Bucha
Sr. M. Helen Rosarie Arakelian
Sr. M. Helena Therese of St. Joseph Horan
Sr. M. Hope Therese Angeline Maring
Sr. M. Jacqueline Joseph Wagner
Sr. M. James Teresa of the Holy Angels Weiss
Sr. M. Jeanette David Lindsay
Sr. M. Jeanne Francis Haley
Sr. M. Joachim Anne Ferenchak

Sr. M. Joan Rita Anne Jennings
Sr. M. Joseph Augustine Thornley
Sr. M. Joseph Catherine De Lourdes Raymond
Sr. M. Joseph Deirdre Tymon
Sr. M. Joseph Jude of the Holy Face Spring
Sr. M. Joseph Marie Maloney
Sr. M. Julie of St. Joseph McCarthy
Sr. M. Kathleen John Immaculate McLinden
Sr. M. Kevin Patricia of St. Joseph O'Brien
Sr. M. Kevin Patricia of the Holy Angels Lynch
Sr. M. Lois Joseph Baniewicz
Sr. M. Madeline Angeline Fasano
Sr. M. Margaret Edward of All Saints Costello
Mother M. Mark Louis Anne Randall
Sr. M. Matthew James of All Saints Gay
Sr. M. Michelle Anne Reho
Sr. M. Michelle of All Saints Moore
Sr. M. Patricia Michael Sweeney
Sr. M. Patricia of the Queen of Carmel Markey
Sr. M. Patricia Treasa O'Callaghan
Sr. M. Patrick Michael De Lourdes Kane
Sr. M. Patrick of the Assumption Traynor
Sr. M. Paul Anthony Videtich
Sr. M. Peter Lillian Angeline DiMaria
Sr. M. Philip Ann of All Saints Bowden
Sr. M. Philomena Anne of Divine Mercy Schill
Sr. M. Raphael Peregrine of the Holy Face Schmitz
Sr. M. Regina Monique Molner
Sr. M. Richard of Jesus Ryan
Sr. M. Robert Anthony of the Holy Angels Didas
Sr. M. Rose of the Sacred Heart Spencer
Sr. M. Seán Damien Flynn
Sr. M. Sean William of All Saints O'Brien
Sr. M. Shawn Bernadette Flynn
Sr. M. Shawn Bernard of the Holy Spirit Daniel
Sr. M. Sylvester of the Holy Angels Thomas
Sr. M. Teresa Kathleen Dominick
Sr. M. Teresa Lucy Bolognese
Sr. M. Teresa Monica Toussaint
Sr. M. Teresa Robert Nekoranec
Sr. M. Teresa Stephen Pereira
Sr. M. Theresa of the Eucharist Pham
Sr. M. Therese Eileen of All Saints Mulvaney
Sr. M. Therese of Jesus Harpur
Sr. M. Therese of the Child Jesus Foley
Sr. M. Therese Suzanne Rankin
Sr. M. Timothy Anne Iovannone
Sr. M. Titus Joseph Ramsbottom
Sr. M. Veronica Robert Bien
Sr. M. Veronica Therese De Lourdes Charlton
Sr. M. Virginia Aloysius Russo
Sr. M. Winifred Angeline Jordan
Sr. M. Xavier Frances Marchiony
Sr. Margaret Mary Boyle
Sr. Margaret Therese Marie Jackson
Sr. Maria Agnes O'Leary
Sr. Maria Robert Mullen
Sr. Maria Therese Healy
Sr. Marie Richard Carmel Brusca
Sr. Mary Ann Immaculate Wasilko
Sr. Mary Anne Dennehy
Sr. Mary Elizabeth Sheffer
Sr. Mary Josephine Crowe
Sr. Mary of Jesus O'Donovan
Sr. Mary Paul of the Eucharist Tenneson
Sr. Mary Robert of the Infant Jesus Romano
Sr. Mary Rose Heery
Sr. Mary Suzanne Sapa
Sr. Mary Vianney Dinh
Sr. Maureen Carroll
Sr. Maureen de Lourdes McDonough
Sr. Maureen Elizabeth Doonan
Sr. Maureen Murray
Sr. Maureen Paul Angeline Sullivan
Sr. Maureen Rochford
Sr. Michael Mary Campbell
Sr. Patricia Brancaccio
Sr. Patricia Margaret Rawdon
Sr. Pauline Brecanier
Sr. Pauline Ross
Sr. Suzanne Marie Ronan
Sr. Theresa Margaret Cave
Sr. Theresa Marie Pfeffer
Sr. Therese Mary Bukowski

Postulants

Sr. Doris Benitez
Sr. Sharon Mullin
Sr. Morgan Mondello

Foundations

Year	Name of Facility	Location	Status
1929	St. Elizabeth	New York, NY	closed 1931 [1]
1931	St. Patrick's Home	New York, NY	
1934	Mount Carmel Villa	New York, NY	closed 1935 [2]
1935	Mount Carmel Home	New York, NY	closed 1981 [3]
1936	Mount Carmel Villa	Philadelphia, PA	closed 1953 [4]
1937	Sacred Heart Manor	Philadelphia, PA	closed 2009
1938	St. Agnes Residence	Philadelphia, PA	closed 1957
1938	St. Joseph's Home	Staten Island, NY	closed 1955
1939	Catholic Memorial Home	Fall River, MA	withdrew 2003
1941	Our Lady of Providence Seminary	Providence, RI	withdrew 1950
1941	St. Leo's Abbey	St. Leo, FL	withdrew 1952
1941	Curé of Ars Hospice	Brakney, PA	closed 1949 [5]
1943	St. Joseph's Seminary	Dunwoodie, NY	withdrew 1969
1943	Cathedral Faculty House	New York, NY	withdrew 1969
1943	St. Luke's Infirmary	Centralia, WA	withdrew 1945
1944	Bishop's Residence	Albany, NY	withdrew 1977
1945	Diocesan Mission House	Chicago, IL	withdrew 1948
1945	Our Lady's Haven	Fairhaven, MA	withdrew 1985
1945	St. Mary's Day Nursery	Chicago, IL	closed 1955
1947	Episcopal Residence	Trenton, NY	withdrew 1959
1947	St. Teresa's Motherhouse and Novitiate	Germantown, NY	
1948	St. Raphael's Home	Columbus, OH	closed 2005 [6]
1949	St. Rita's Home	Columbus, OH	closed 2005 [7]
1949	St. Margaret Mary House	Washington, DC	closed 1957 [8]
1949	St. Francis Home	Laconia, NH	withdrew 1985
1949	Mount Carmel Home	Manchester, NH	withdrew 1985
1949	Carmel Manor	Fort Thomas, KY	
1950	Bishop's Residence	Columbus, OH	withdrew 1957
1950	Sacred Heart Home	Chicago, IL	closed 1972
1951	Villa Maria	North Miami, FL	withdrew 1958
1951	St. Joseph's Manor	St. Petersburg, FL	closed 1958
1951	St. Mary's Home	Youngstown, OH	closed 1972
1952	Mary Manning Walsh	New York, NY	closed 1969 [9]

1953	St. Patrick's Manor	Boston, MA	closed 1970 [10]
1954	Marian Manor	South Boston, MA	
1954	Welty Memorial Home	Wheeling, WV	withdrew 1961
1954	Mater Christi Seminary	Albany, NY	closed 1972 [11]
1955	Kahl Memorial Home	Davenport, IA	closed 2012 [12]
1955	Josephine Baird Home	New York, NY	closed 1972
1955	Carmel Hall	Detroit, MI	withdrew 1979
1957	Carroll Manor	Hyattsville, MD	withdrew 1991
1958	St. Ann's Home	Dover, NH	withdrew 1997
1960	Madonna Residence	Brooklyn, NY	closed 1995
1960	St. Joseph's Manor	Trumbull, CT	withdrew 2006
1961	Lourdes Residence	West Palm Beach, FL	closed 1975 [13]
1962	St. Margaret Hall	Cincinnati, OH	
1964	Bethania	Dunoon, Scotland	withdrew 1974
1965	Ferncliff	Rhinebeck, NY	withdrew 2009
1965	Our Lady's Manor	Dalkey, Dublin, Ireland	
1965	Garvey Manor	Hollidaysburg, PA	
1965	St. Patrick's Residence	Joliet, IL	closed 1989 [14]
1965	The Pennsylvania/Lourdes Residence	West Palm Beach, FL	closed 1998
1969	Mary Manning Walsh Home	New York, NY	
1969	Mount Carmel Nursing Home	Manchester, NH	withdrew 1997
1970	St. Patrick's Manor	Framingham, MA	
1971	Ozanam Hall	Bayside, NY	
1971	St. Joseph's Nursing Home	Utica, NY	withdrew 2014
1973	Villa Teresa	Harrisburg, PA	closed 2005
1974	Carmel Richmond	Staten Island, NY	
1974	Teresian House	Albany, NY	
1974	Little Flower Manor	Wilkes-Barre, PA	
1980	Lourdes–Noreen McKeen Residence	West Palm Beach, FL	
1989	St. Patrick's Residence	Naperville, IL	
1995	Carmel Terrace	Framingham, MA	
1999	The Villas at St. Thérèse	Columbus, OH	
2005	Mother Angeline McCrory Manor	Columbus, OH	
2013	Mount Carmel Care Center	Lenox, MA	

1. Residents moved to St. Patrick's Home.
2. Residents moved to Mount Carmel Home.
3. Could not be brought up to code.
4. Became too small.
5. Closed by the diocese.
6. Residents moved to Mother Angeline McCrory Manor.
7. Residents moved to Mother Angeline McCrory Manor.
8. Residents moved to Carroll Manor.
9. Residents moved to Mary Manning Walsh Home.
10. New facility of the same name opened that year in Framingham, residents moved there.
11. Closed by the diocese.
12. Residents moved to a new facility with the same name.
13. Combined with the Pennsylvania into new Lourdes–Noreen McKeen Residence in 1980.
14. Residents transferred to new facility in Naperville, IL.

Awards

Mother Angeline Teresa
Papal award of Pro Ecclesia et Pontifice Medal (1961)
National Award of Honor from the American Association of Homes for the Aging (1969)
Honorary Degree of Humane Letters, Siena College (1970)
Honorary Degree of Humane Letters, Manhattan College (1970)
Papal award of Benemerenti Medal (1978)

Mother Suzanne
Caritas Medal, St. John's University (2004)

Mother Bernadette
Honorary Doctor of Laws, University of Bridgeport (1969)
Honorary Doctor of Laws, Sacred Heart University (1974)

Carmelite Sisters
Panis Vitae Award (1995)
Annual Award of the Hospital Apostolate Archdiocese of New York (1995)
Cardinal Cooke Right to Life Award (1996)
Alfred E. Smith Memorial Foundation Award for Health Care (1997)
St. Louise de Marilla Award (2005)
Msgr. James J. Murray Memorial Award (2011)

Bibliography

Carmelite Sisters for the Aged and Infirm, The. Strasbourg, France: Editions du Signe, 2000.
Farren, Suzy. *A Call to Care*. St Louis, MO: Scholin Brothers Printing, 1996.
Lopez, Michael. "Divine Calling." *Times Union*. April 16, 2000.
Mead, Rev. Jude, C.P. *The Servant of God Mother M. Angeline*. Petersham, MA: St. Bede's Publications, 1989.
Reis, Sr. M. Gabriel, O.Carm. *Seed Scattered and Sown*. Privately printed, 1991.
Tschanz, Anne. "Venerable Mary Angeline Teresa McCrory – Daughter of Carmel, Mother to the Aged." *Religious Life*. July/August 2014.
Wisely, Mother M. Bernadette de Lourdes, O.Carm. *Where Somebody Cares*. New York, NY: G. P. Putnam's Sons, 1959.
————. *Woman of Faith*. 1984.